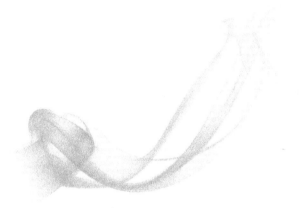

Chasing Rainbows

My Triumph Over Ovarian Cancer

Luci Berardi

Chasing Rainbows: My Triumph Over Ovarian Cancer

© Copyright 2013 Luci Berardi

All rights reserved. No part of this book may be reproduced or distributed in any form or by any means (written, electronic, mechanical, recording, photocopy or otherwise) or stored in a database or retrieval system, without the prior written permission of the author or publisher, except in the case of brief quotations embodied in critical articles and reviews.

Disclaimer
The information written in this book is not intended to diagnose, treat or prevent disease. Nothing in this book should be viewed as a substitute or replacement for competent medical care. Please consult your physician prior to undertaking any changes to your diet or exercise regimen.

> Books may be purchased in quantity and/or special sales by contacting the author or publisher at: YogiLuci@yahoo.com

Cover and Interior Design: NZ Graphics (Nick Zelinger)
Editing: Judith Briles (The BookShepherd), and John Maling (Editing By John)
Publisher: Triumphant Press

Library of Congress Control Number: 2012941749

ISBN-13: 978-0-9856668-0-4

10 9 8 7 6 5 4 3 2 1

1. Memoir   2. Ovarian Cancer   3. Cancer Recovery   4. Holistic Medicine

First Edition

Printed in the United States of America

Acknowledgments

To the love of my life, Todd

Thank you for walking this journey with me. Through the fears, pain, and anger, you remained supportive and strong. You are my rock. I love you.

Mo Anam Cara

To my Mother

You are the epitome of the unconditional love shared between a mother and child. Your love, support and strength were instrumental in my ability to keep fighting. You are an amazing woman and I'm proud to call you "Mom."

To Aunt Lucy

When I was unable to care for myself, you were right there for me. You remained positive and supportive for my sake, in spite of all the uncertainties. For this I am forever grateful. You are truly stronger than you think.

To my mother-in-law, Sue

I offer my heartfelt gratitude to you for sharing your wisdom, knowledge and your own cancer experience with me. I cherish the special bond we share and thank you for the continuous healings and cleansings you performed on me; both on the spiritual and astral levels.

To my Father-in-Law, Burton

From chauffeur to chef to companion and shopping buddy, you were a tremendous help. Your sense of humor and manner was such a welcomed distraction. Thank you for the many hats you wore and reminding me of the importance of laughter.

To my BFF, Rita

Our friendship is like that of no other. I am so grateful to have you in my life and I can't thank you enough for being by my side during the greatest fight of my life. During my darkest moments, you always knew what to say and your wisdom helped get me through it.

To Dr. Mary Jo Schmitz

Your knowledge, experience and aggressiveness saved my life. You are truly an angel of God. Thank you.

To my Father

Although you no longer walk this earth with us, your spiritual presence was unmistakable. Thank you for being with me through this fight. "Your little girl."

Although I can't individually name every person, I would like to thank my family, friends, co-workers and acquaintances for your love, support and prayers during my fight. You have each touched my life in a special way and I will forever hold your kindnesses within my heart.

Foreword

My title, *Chasing Rainbows*, came from my husband, Todd, who was ever observant on my compulsiveness seeking other possible avenues of help with my affliction late in my treatment regimen. I was desperate—why not find my own rainbow?

They ranged from conventional medicine, alternative therapies and the spiritual. In the end, I found they all played an essential role in my successful campaign to become, and remain once again, cancer-free. And they also led to a new lease on life—for my beloved husband, Todd, and myself.

If you are reading *Chasing Rainbows*, it is possible you have been recently diagnosed with ovarian cancer or you know a friend or family member who is already in that life or death fight. I was compelled to write this book ... My intention? To provide fellow cancer fighters with the weapons of hope and alternative therapies after diagnosis and during and after active treatment.

Although many cancer treatments are similar, my focus is primarily on ovarian cancer. Ovarian cancer is the deadliest of the female cancers, due in part to the often late diagnosis and advanced staging afterwards when finally diagnosed.

Some of the most common warning signs of ovarian cancer are bloating, feeling full after eating—even small amounts—bleeding and pain during intercourse. What makes this cancer hard to diagnose is that the warning signs often mimic pre-menstrual symptoms. Many women who are diagnosed with ovarian cancer are surprised by the diagnosis. Stunned and shocked would be a better description. Their responses were similar to mine:

I was in fairly good health, exercised, and ate well. How could this happen?

Unfortunately, there is still no accurate testing for this cancer as I share my story with you.

If there is one thing I hope every reader takes away from my experience, it is this: you must be your own advocate. Do not just accept what a physician tells you; listen to your body. Make sure you ask questions, and if something doesn't feel right, be sure to share your concerns with your physician or get a second opinion.

If you have been diagnosed with cancer, I'm sure you too have asked the same question: "How could this have happened to me?" I know I did. There are many different scenarios to this question. There may be family history, a genetic mutation to the BRCA-1 gene mutation, as in my case, or to BRCA-2, and reasons that science still cannot answer. The important thing to remember is not to get caught up in trying to be a detective to solve this so-called mystery. Your energy and strength will better serve you if you focus on fighting this disease. I want to help you and your loved ones by sharing with you my journey, to fight this fight with every stitch in the fabric of your soul.

As you embark on this journey, as a cancer fighter or a caregiver, there are a few things I need to share with you:

> First, there will be times during this fight which will be more difficult than others; never lose hope. There are survivors of this disease and you have every chance to be one.

> Secondly, know that you will meet such wonderful people on this path, people who will forever change the way you look at life. Special bonds will be formed among fellow cancer fighters and survivors. Once you are one, you'll know exactly what I mean.

> We all want—hope—to beat this disease, to go back to our once "normal" life, and not die. We are all frightened, and the unconditional caring and hope we feel among other fighters and survivors will provide a source of comfort.

> Thirdly, know it's okay to ask for help. Letting others do things for you is okay.

This was life-changing for me personally. I am a "need to be in control" personality type. But I am here to say cancer is very humbling. You will be tired and exhausted. Don't worry about feeling badly about asking for help. One thing I discovered was that people really wanted to reach out and help, but they didn't know how. I think the asking gave them a sense of purpose to participate and not feel so helpless.

And finally, know this disease, in one way or another, touches everyone … whether you are the fighter or the caregiver or a loved one. Each one of us has our own struggle in the battle against ovarian cancer.

1

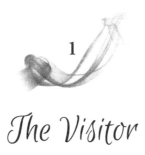

The Visitor

"I can't die. I'm only 42 years old."

Evening had just set in. As I peered outside my window, the city lights lit up the evening sky with the silhouette of the Rocky Mountains faintly visible in the far distance. The sky was clear. How long will it be? Were they able to reach him? Did he know how serious this was? Time seemed to stand still as my gaze shifted from the window to the door.

I was startled by a faint knock at the door. The time was 10:30 p.m., my heart began to beat faster. I sat up quickly in my bed and said, "Come in."

"Lucille?" he asked.

I knew who it was. "Yes, Father, please come in."

Entering my room, he closed the door behind him. He walked over to the side of my hospital bed and extended his hand to me. "Hello, Lucille, I'm Father John."

"Thank you for coming, Father."

"I apologize for coming so late; I was helping a family with funeral arrangements."

"No need to apologize; thank you for coming."

He softly asked, "How may I help you, Lucille?"

Trying to hold in my emotion, I replied, "Well, Father, I was just diagnosed with ovarian cancer and I am scheduled for surgery tomorrow morning. I would like to receive the Sacrament of Reconciliation and Communion and the Anointing of the Sick."

He pulled a chair from the desk and came to sit at the side of my bed. "I would be happy to."

This was going to be the fight of my life, for my life.

Taking out his prayer book he began to pray over me. After confession, he performed the blessing over the host and offered me Communion. Father John then proceeded with the anointing. He placed oil in my palms and continued to pray over me. Blessing me he then made the sign of the cross over my head and placed his hand on my head. Just before he left the room, he said, "God Bless you." I felt comfort and calmness at that Moment and a sense of peace within.

I remember sitting there in bed saying in my mind, "It's going to be okay."

There were so many random thoughts that ran through my mind that night as I had an ongoing conversation with myself.

"You are strong Lucille and you will make it through this."

"I can't die; I'm only 42 years old."

"I have only been married to Todd for two years. Our life together has just begun."

"There was no way that my mother was going to bury her daughter."

This was going to be the fight of my life for my life. I finally felt ready and up to the challenge. Feeling the sense of peace that enveloped me when Father John had left the room, I found myself becoming sleepy. I reached over and turned off the lights.

Mom's Take

When this was happening, it was like a nightmare, always worrying something more would be found.

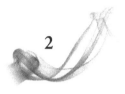

2

The Symptoms

***The nurse told me that the doctor didn't have
the answer for "This."***

On July 6, 2010, I noticed my right rib had what seemed to be a bump or bulge. I was sure this was not something that had always been there. In fact, every ounce of my being told me that it didn't belong on my body! That bumpy bulge rudely interrupted my sleep one night. Since I can remember, I've been a stomach sleeper and my right rib began to bother me when I would lie on it. My first thought was that I might have done something during one of my yoga practices, so I didn't get alarmed; I thought I would just keep an eye on it.

Todd and I both work long weeks and love our weekends. We enjoy our Saturdays, spending time together in bed relishing our amazing fortune in finding each other.

The Symptoms

What started out to be a normal weekend morning for Todd and I turned out quite differently. This was the first sign that something was wrong. During our love making, I had such an unbearable pain within my pelvic region, we were forced to stop. The sensation of pain was nothing I had ever felt before. The date was July 31, 2010.

On Monday morning, I called my gynecologist for an appointment. I was able to get an appointment the same day. I informed him of my symptoms of severe pain during intercourse, being bloated in the stomach and also told him about this "bump" on my rib. Performing a pelvic exam, he recommended I come back for a trans-vaginal ultrasound the next day.

On Tuesday, August 3, 2010, I had a trans-vaginal ultrasound. The procedure was uneventful and only took 15 minutes. I remember the tech telling me that my ovaries looked normal and added that my doctor would read the report and would get back to me.

On Friday, I received a call from my doctor's nurse with the findings. She told me there seemed to be the remains of a hemorragic cyst on the right ovary and fluid in the abdominal region. The doctor had recommended a course of treatment using birth control pills for 30 days. The birth control pills were being prescribed to see if this would get rid of the cyst. Picking up my prescription, I began my 30 day regimen on Sunday.

Thinking I was dealing with a cyst, I again turned my attention to the bumpy bulge on my rib which had remained unchanged. On Monday, August 16, I called my primary physician and learned he was out of town. His office scheduled me with the physician's assistant on staff who evaluated the area and recommended I take Ibuprofen three to four times a day for the discomfort. Ibuprofen did nothing—the discomfort persisted. Three days later I called back and set up an appointment with my primary care physician for the end of the month, August 30.

Todd and I had planned a long weekend getaway to San Diego the last week of August. During our mini vacation, we again attempted intercourse, being the first time since the episode at the end of July. Horrific pain screamed through my body. We could not finish what we started. My mind searched for a reason for the pain. My first thought was fibroids, since I had had one five years previously and had to have surgery to remove it from the uterine wall.

Todd was getting concerned and came with me to my scheduled appointment with my primary care physician. While he evaluated my rib area, I told him that I was seeing my gynecologist for some female issues. He said, "These two things are totally unrelated." In his opinion, I had somehow damaged the cartilage on my ribcage. A topical pain cream was prescribed that he wanted me to use for two weeks to see if there would be any improvement. A day or two passed and I began to wonder why he hadn't taken an x-ray of my rib. I called back to his office and asked to be scheduled for one. His medical assistant said an x-ray would most likely not show anything and the doctor wanted to wait on the findings from my gynecologist. I reluctantly agreed to wait.

I pleaded with her and told her. "I know my body and there is something wrong."

On September 9, I returned to my gynecologist for a repeat transvaginal ultrasound. The results were similar to the first one, done the previous month. "Nothing out of the ordinary," was relayed to me. The following week, my gynecologist's nurse called and told me the cyst appeared to be gone, but there was still fluid in my abdominal region. Fibroids were present, measuring in millimeters.

"Why is there still fluid in the abdominal region?" I asked. She told me the doctor did not have an answer for this. His recommendation was to have a hysterectomy.

"A WHAT????? I'm 42 years old and this seems quite extreme for a few fibroids that don't seem to be causing the issue." I finished the call, telling her that I would need to think about this and that this recommendation seemed very radical.

I began to inquire about pre-menopausal symptoms and treatments. After all, I was 42—maybe I was starting menopause. The symptoms that I had been experiencing had remained unchanged with one exception. During September I began to notice during my yoga practice, whenever I went into an inverted pose like Down Dog,

I began to cough. It was as though I couldn't take in deep breaths without wanting to cough and had a feeling of heaviness in my upper back. Is this what happens at 42 … everything falls apart?

As many of us know too well … the Internet is an awesome tool for searching out different things, but it too can provide too many possible answers to problems. As a result, my searches made me a wreck. I began to think I had every disease that was out there.

Todd has chided me many times in the past, because I tend to obsess over things and can over-react. One condition which surfaced during my many searches was Congestive Heart Failure. Since I have Mitral Valve Prolapse (MVP) with severe regurgitation, I thought perhaps I was beginning to develop fluid retention in my lungs due to the MVP. I have been under the care of a cardiologist for many years and I was well aware I would more than likely need to have a valve repair surgery sometime in the future.

On Monday, October 4, 2010, I placed another call to my primary care physician and asked to leave a message for him—that I would like to have a CT or MRI done. Shortly after leaving the message, I received a call from the doctor's triage nurse. She told me I would need to come in to see the doctor before my procedure could be scheduled. I told her I had been in twice and no one would take an x-ray. I repeated my symptoms of bloating, coughing, and the pressure in my upper back. I became emotional and began crying. I pleaded with her and told

The Symptoms

her, "I know my body and there is something wrong, but I don't know what it is. I guess I'll end up in the ER if it gets bad enough." She told me she would discuss this with the doctor and call me back. She did call back and scheduled me for a visit with another doctor—this time with a GI specialist.

Wednesday, October 6, found me at the GI specialist. I explained my symptoms to the nurse practitioner and also told her about my "bump." She commented that their focus is on the GI tract and not on the rib. After this consultation, her recommendation was to have an Endoscopy. Additionally, she recommended I have a special panel of blood work drawn to rule out H-pylori, a bacteria found in the stomach. This could cause additional problems, even cancer if not treated. I was brought to the scheduling coordinator and scheduled for an Endoscopy a month later—November 15.

The next day was Thursday, October 7. I headed to Utah to see my family. My mother, my Aunt Lucy (my mother's sister), my two brothers, their wives, and my niece Brooklyn and nephew Braxton all live in Utah. Having no children of my own, Brooklyn and Braxton are the next best thing. I think of them as my own and I just love visiting them. Getting to Utah three to four times a year was a priority for me. Although flight time was less than an hour away.

During this visit, the pain across my upper back and into my upper chest became more pronounced. It had become difficult to sleep comfortably at night. My younger brother Jerry is married to Christie, a nurse. I showed her my rib. She said flat out, "This is not normal, you need to get that looked at."

At the same time, I confided to my Mom what had been going on with my health.

Following Christie's advice and my mother's concern, I tried to get an appointment with my mother's doctor for an x-ray. None were available. I didn't think it was urgent enough to go to the ER in Utah, since I would be back home in Colorado in a few days.

Todd's Take

I'm one who refuses to see an M.D., unless the bleeding continues after duct tape has been applied. So when Luci was scheduling appointments with the various doctors, I made the assumption that they were in complete control. How sadly mistaken I was. Through the various visits, I tended to side with them and considered Luci's observations of her own body an obsession. Every time she mentioned a new pain or discomfort I told her, "Wait and see; these were qualified doctors after all."

The Symptoms

I had accompanied her to our primary care physician and his initial diagnosis made sense. Luci could have damaged some connective tissue during her Yoga practice. With each continuing diagnosis, she kept me informed. Everything seemed to coincide with typical "female problems." I thought she might be approaching menopause.

I had no idea what was to come. I later came to regret my "wait and see" attitude.

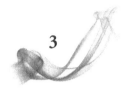

3

Who Am I?

"As with any Italian family, there was more food than you could eat and it was very loud."

I am recently married to a wonderful man, Todd. We have two dogs; Tara, a Weimaraner and Rafferty, a Lab-Shepherd mix who are our "children." Todd and I just celebrated our second wedding anniversary in July.

Professionally, I am a Practice Manager for a periodontal and implant practice where I have worked for the past 17 years. Todd is self-employed which allows us a lot of flexibility in scheduling short trips. Weekend getaways we planned several times a year—a two-week vacation somewhere abroad is something we both plan and look forward to. During the summer months the beauty of Colorado beckons us. We hit the highways and back roads on our Harley-Davidson. Our life is good.

Todd and I met each other in 1997 through our mutual friends, Aimee and Chris, who lived across the street from me. At that time, I was married to a musician. Todd first met Chris through the Colorado Air National Guard and then they worked together in the HVAC industry. Throughout the next several years, Todd and I would see one another at gatherings where Aimee and Chris were. Beneath it, there always seemed to be an unspoken attraction between the two of us. We just didn't know to what extent it would lead.

The musician and I stopped "making music" in 2002. We had such different views on where we saw our lives going and had fewer and fewer things in common. I kept this to myself, and never let on to any of my friends or family of my problems. Our work schedules were completely opposite, which created more sour notes and contributed to our difficulties. Aimee's house became my retreat on the weekends. There comes a time in one's life when you need to stop worrying about what others may think or say. You need to listen to your inner voice and do what is right for you. I did, and my first marriage ended in divorce. The year was 2004.

I am a believer in fate and I believe there are no coincidences in life. It wouldn't be for another six years that I would fully understand why Todd and I were destined to be together.

I was 42 years old when I was diagnosed with ovarian cancer. The resulting tsunami almost drowned us in its breadth. I thought of myself as a fairly healthy person. As a registered yoga instructor, I had been practicing yoga for over 12 years. Rarely, if ever, did I eat any "white" foods; loved all type of vegetables; and practiced meditation. Once in a while, I would eat meat, and I consumed quite a bit of dairy foods. My weakness? I loved chocolate. Let me re-phrase this, I was a chocoholic. I never gave a second thought to eating chocolate at 6:30 in the morning. Most evenings, a glass of wine was enjoyed as I unwound from my day.

I never really gave this much thought until I was faced with the fight of my life to fight for my life.

Weight challenges weren't on my dance card. Now to some of you, I know you must be thinking "Lucky you, if I just look at a piece of cake, I gain ten pounds." Well, I'm the one who developed cancer, so now who's the lucky one? It wasn't until after my diagnosis that I began to do research and found out how refined sugars found in many desserts and candies actually assist cancer growth. These cancer cells could not have wished for a better host. I became a breeder for them.

It's funny how when you are faced with a life-threatening situation, you look back and ponder your childhood and how so many things in the past had a direct impact of who you are today. I was born to Patricia and Anthony

Berardi in May of 1968 in Brooklyn, New York. In following with our proud Italian family tradition, I was named after my father's mother, my nana, Lucille Berardi. My brothers were named after our grandfathers. I was the second of three children. My older brother Frank is just eleven months older than me and Jerry is five years my junior.

We were raised in what I will call a traditional Catholic Italian family setting. Whether it was a holiday, birthday, communion or just a Sunday dinner, my aunts, uncles, grandmothers and cousins always surrounded me. As with any Italian gathering, there was more food than you could eat and it was very loud. As I reflect back, I am so grateful for my childhood and the memories of this period of my life, surrounded by all our relatives for every occasion.

My nana and my mother were the biggest influences on me. Both provided me with the strength and determination to fight for what I believed in and never accept anything less. I never really gave this much thought until I was faced with the fight *of* my life to fight *for* my life.

The closeness I had with my family as a child is still a very important part of my life.

The lessons I learned from my nana and lessons I continue to learn from my mother, along with the love and support I received from my family and my friends during my illness helped me through my battle with ovarian cancer. For this I am forever indebted to them.

Mom's Take

What a wonderful weekend we were going to have October 2010. My daughter Lucille came to visit us in Utah every few months. She loved to come and visit with her niece Brooklyn and nephew Braxton. We had a great visit, although she wasn't feeling too well the entire visit. She had what seemed to be a chronic cough and didn't look herself. She said she was having trouble breathing. We all thought it was due to the faulty heart valve she has.

Well, the weekend ended and she left to go home. Later that evening her husband Todd called us that they went to the emergency room because Luci couldn't breathe. They aspirated a great deal of liquid from her lungs. Naturally we thought it might be congestive heart failure. They kept her overnight to do various tests. Now the waiting game began …

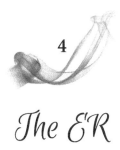

4

The ER

"I felt for a moment I must be in a dream."

I flew back to Colorado from Utah on Sunday, October 10. Todd and I had dinner plans with our neighbors, Ray and Sherri, that evening.

Ray and Sherri came into our lives when Todd saw Ray shoveling snow at the base of his driveway. The only use for a shovel when living in the mountains is to clear off your deck or dig your way to the snowplow. I use the word "driveway" loosely when describing Ray's driveway. It best resembles an uphill access dirt road with two switchbacks and a 200 foot incline. Their home sits about 70 yards above our home on the hill.

Todd had just finished plowing our driveway with his ATV. He drove over to Ray who was diligently shoveling snow. "That's a good way to give yourself a heart attack.

I'd be happy to plow your drive for you." Ray smiled and said, "Oh no, that's alright. I don't want to bother you."

For Todd, that was as good as an invitation. Todd came home and told me to get my coat and boots on. "I just met our new neighbors and they've invited us up for coffee." From then on, our friendship continued to grow.

Over the next several years, the four of us spent a lot of time together. We would spend snowy nights and summer nights at each other's house playing cards or dominoes. We began to jokingly reference each home as "Upstairs" and "Downstairs."

For Todd and I, not only had our homes become an extension, Ray and Sherri were our extended family. Although not feeling good, I looked forward to seeing them.

As I was leaving the parking lot where I had parked my car, something came over me. I can't fully explain what it was, but it was clear and imperative. My head and body were telling me that I needed to go to the ER tonight! As I drove from the airport, I began to merge over to the right lane to take the exit which would get me to Rose Hospital. This is where my cardiologist's office was and in my mind, all my symptoms were related to my heart. Then a change of destination. I felt I was being told to keep driving towards home and not to exit here for the hospital.

I was hesitant at first to call Todd, because I thought he was going to say I was over-reacting and reading too much into my host of symptoms. Finally I called him as I was on the brink of crying. When he answered, I told him I needed to go the doctor right away.

I kept thinking this can't be real; how could this be?

"What's wrong?"

I began to cry. "I don't know, but there *is* something wrong."

"Do you need to go to the ER right now? I can meet you there—or can you come home first and we can drive to the ER together?"

I did not feel I was in imminent danger so I went home and picked him up. Dinner with Ray and Sherri was cancelled.

As Todd drove us to Denver, he asked which hospital he should go to. I said Rose since that's where my cardiologist is. He said, "Swedish is closer; I know exactly where the ER entrance is." We arrived at Swedish Medical Center around 6 p.m.

Upon filling out the intake form, I was rushed back immediately due to the symptoms of heaviness in the chest and difficulty breathing. In a matter of minutes, I was undressed, covered with wires, on oxygen, and a pulse meter was placed on my index finger.

The ER doctor came in and ordered an EKG and a chest x-ray. Shortly thereafter he returned and said there is definitely something going on in the lung area, and he ordered a CT scan of the chest and abdomen.

About 45 minutes later he came back into the room, leaned up against the counter, his right leg crossed over his left, and his arms crossed. Neither Todd nor I were prepared or expecting the next words out of his mouth. "Based on the results of your CT scan it appears you have cancer."

A numbing sensation came over my entire body. I felt my heartbeat begin to increase. I felt for a Moment that I was in a dream. I don't recall if I said anything back to him.

"At this point we are unsure what form of cancer it is. It has spread throughout your abdomen. It would be like taking a paint brush and flicking it."

He went on to say there is fluid in the pleura sack in the right lung. This is what's causing the heaviness in your chest. He added that a call has been placed to the pulmonary doctor on call, and he left the room.

I kept thinking that this can't be real; how could this be?

I was sure it was my heart. I looked over at Todd. His eyes were filling up with tears. Maybe there was a mistake. I called my mother and told her I was in the ER and they weren't sure what exactly was wrong; tests were still being run. I couldn't bear to even say the "C" word to her.

I then called my best friend, Rita. This was about 9:30 pm. She and Michael had just finished dinner and were strolling along Pearl Street Mall in Boulder. After hearing the news, she immediately said they were on their way down.

It's amazing how the mind works. I suspect its behavior is to protect us. If you can stay busy, you can step out of reality and for a period of time you don't have to face it. I thought, "Oh my God, I'm supposed to teach yoga tomorrow."

Thank goodness for the Blackberry. I sent a text message to the studio owner to let her know that I was in the ER and I would not be able to teach tomorrow morning. I also sent an email to my friend Jeannine who also taught yoga at the same studio and asked her if she could cover my class. Thankfully she responded immediately. I also decided to send a text to the other studio where I taught on Thursday evenings.

I knew I wouldn't be going home for several days. During this time of taking care of business, Todd was busy on his phone calling his parents and our closest friends. We were on autopilot.

After what seemed like hours, the pulmonologist came into the room. He explained to Todd and me that I had a Pleura Effusion. This occurs when fluid builds up in the area between the rib and the pleura sac that surrounds the lung. He recommended draining the fluid. This would provide relief of the pressure I was experiencing in the chest and with breathing. He further explained that the procedure would involve numbing an area on my upper back and inserting a needle to remove the fluid.

Due to the amount of fluid in the pleura sac, he wanted to have the fluid drained by gravity versus manually extracting it. Because the fluid had been building up over a period of time, the lung had been "pushed" upward and compressed by my rib. Removing it quickly would cause the lung to inflate. The result for me would be a severe, uncontrollable coughing attack, which would be very uncomfortable.

Consenting to the procedure seemed like an obvious thing to do. As I was being prepped for this procedure, the doctor recommended I sit on the side of the bed with my legs hanging over the side. I was to cross my arms, rest them on the stainless steel surgical cart and place my head down on top of my crossed arms. A pillow was added for additional comfort.

I was told, "Take a deep breath. You will now feel a small poke," and he injected the lidocaine to numb the area in my back. A few moments later, he began the procedure that would release the fluid—the fluid that shouldn't be around my lung.

I was so happy to see Rita and Michael who came into my room just a few minutes later. I remember a smile spreading across my face. Suddenly I began to get very hot and sweaty and nauseous. "I'm going to get sick."

The doctor immediately ordered an IV for an anti-nausea medication. The nurse administered the drug and the results were almost immediate. Rita placed a baggie of ice on the nape of my neck and gently caressed my head, moving my hair from my face and blowing on my forehead to comfort me. Time passed slowly.

The procedure took about 25 minutes. I started to notice I was able to breathe more deeply. As I began to take longer, deeper breaths, I started coughing. The doctor felt I had had enough. I was exhausted. Two liters of fluid were removed from the pleura restricting my right lung. I couldn't believe it. I remember telling the doctor about my heart condition and asking if he thought this could be related. "Possibly, but we will send it to the lab for testing," was his response.

He also commented that the color of the fluid looked good and had no sign of blood in it. He said something about "good body fluids look like beer." That observation gave me a sense of relief.

For the first time since being admitted to the ER, Todd smiled. Maybe there was a chance that I didn't have cancer and it was really something with my heart. Looking back now, I don't think the doctor had the heart to tell us any further devastating news.

The ER doctor came back in and told me I was being admitted shortly after the completion of the pleural drainage. It was approaching midnight and none of us knew what to expect next.

Todd's Take

When Luci called me from DIA, I knew something was really wrong. Luci isn't prone to unexplained teary outbursts. When she met me at the bottom of our driveway, I could see she was scared. During the forty minute drive, she recounted the discomfort she had experienced during her trip. Just knowing we were on the way to the ER seemed to calm her.

Based on her symptoms, she was treated immediately as a coronary patient when we arrived. When the x-ray revealed fluid accumulation, we started to discuss the heart surgery—it was earlier than we expected but well within our expectations.

Once the CT scan came back and the ER doc said, "Cancer," I was lost. In my mind, cancer happens to older people, people who smoke and don't take care of themselves. My wife of two years does not have cancer! Look at her! She's young, she practices Yoga religiously, she eats right, she has never smoked and rarely drinks! I'm the guy who survived on buffalo wings, frozen pizza and beer for so many years! This can't be right!

The ER

After the initial shock and immediate denial, Luci wanted to call Rita. We also decided to let our closest friends and family know what was going on. I felt like I was on autopilot, I was making phone calls and explaining what little I knew. Everyone asked the same question, "How did this happen?" After two or three phone calls, it became repetitive. I told everyone I'd keep them updated.

When Michael and Rita arrived, my nerves settled a little. We were not going into this alone!

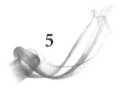

The Diagnosis

"I was determined to maintain a sense of normalcy. In my mind I don't really think the "C" word had sunk in yet."

Time went by in slow motion, stretched out by my many unanswered questions. Around 12:30 a.m., I was finally brought to my new room. Rita and Michael helped settle me in and then left. Todd attempted to sleep on a pull-out sofa next to my bed. Neither of us slept much—nurses were in and out drawing blood and taking vitals into the early dawn.

At 6 a.m., we both woke from cat-napping. Todd decided to go home to check on the dogs and bring me some personal belongings. Arriving back a few hours later, he caught me up on what sounded like a telephone marathon. He had been on the phone from the time he left the hospital, with our families and close friends talking and texting them regarding my status, condition, and any new developments.

In my mind, the "C" word hadn't sunk in yet.

Along with his phone news, he brought my suitcase that was still in the trunk from my return from Utah, along with three different outfits and my laptop. He also thought to bring a favorite picture of us and one of our dogs. I really had no idea how long I was going to be here nor did I know what the plan of attack was. And at that moment, I didn't think the doctors knew either.

Having some of my personal belongings around me helped to create a little more familiar surroundings. If I had to be here, I was not going to be lying around in hospital attire. It felt really good to be able to shower and put some of my normal clothes on again. Off with the gown, on with my lounging yoga attire. Just putting on my own clothes and makeup lifted my spirits. I would later know exactly how important that statement really was …

I was determined to maintain a sense of normalcy. In my mind I don't really think the "C" word had sunk in yet.

It was about 11 a.m. when we first met Dr. Pinzinski, the hospitalist. He came in, checked my vitals and asked how I was feeling. This is what is crazy with my cancer. I really felt fine. I could see that Dr. Pinzinski seemed surprised at how I looked and at my energy level. He said they were looking at several things. He honestly couldn't say whether it was ovarian, gallbladder, stomach or liver cancer. He continued, "I don't believe how well you look and how good you say you feel. You don't have any 'classic symptoms'; your abdomen should be swollen to that of a 20-week pregnant woman." He told me I would be scheduled shortly for a series of tests. As soon as these tests were confirmed and added to the hospital schedule, my nurses would let me know.

So there I sat, just waiting. How could this be happening? All made up and no place to go. Needing a distraction, I turned my attention to my work.

I left work on Thursday, October 7, 2010, as a normal departure, assuming to return on Tuesday, October 12, 2010. That was not to be the case. I have worked for Professional Periodontics & Implant Dentistry for 17 years. During that time, I became the backbone of the practice with exclusive responsibilities for a variety of areas including payroll. I was the only one who knew what needed to be done, and when and how to keep the office running like a clock. After a normal work week, I had left on October 7th for a long weekend with my family in Utah.

Today was Monday, October 11, 2010, and payroll needed to be sent over to our payroll company in time for checks to be printed and mailed for Friday's payroll.

My hospital room became my remote office for the time being. I checked with my administrator and our payroll company to make sure everyone could be paid. I was able to remotely access our office's database to obtain all the necessary information. Technology has come such a long way. Imagine running my office from a hospital bed!

It was necessary to speak with one of the dentists I worked for because there were loose ends that needed to be addressed immediately. And even though I was still considering this a short hospital stay, I had to inform him of my situation just in case my stay would be longer.

After lunch, my nurse informed me I was scheduled tomorrow, Tuesday, October 12, 2010, for an Echocardiogram and a tissue biopsy of the lump on my right rib. There were no dietary restrictions in place for these two appointments. For now, I was able to eat whatever I wanted.

When you're bound to a hospital room, it becomes boring. I've never had to stay overnight in a hospital, but I must say, this hospital had many accommodations for its patients to try to ease this boredom. They offer WIFI, free movies, music, and a pretty wide selection of food choices. I decided to make the best of it by changing my mind-set to that of being in a hotel.

One of the most important decisions I had to make was selecting my meals. What else can you do … it truly is all about your mind-set.

Evening was upon us and Todd was going to spend the night again. Instead, I encouraged him to go home to get some rest. I could see this was beginning to wear on him. After all, tests were scheduled to be done in the morning; there was no reason for him to keep an empty room company.

Tuesday morning arrived as did the technician to escort me to my Echocardiogram. This test was uneventful but very important, in order to rule out any potential heart concerns. My history of having a mitral valve prolapse was a concern for the doctors, especially if surgery was going to be needed. This test took about 20 minutes. I returned to my room around 11 a.m., just in time to place my lunch order.

Around 2 p.m., another technician arrived to escort me to my tissue biopsy. I was wheeled to a surgical outpatient room where I was turned over to the assisting nurse to prep me for the biopsy. The procedure first required local anesthetic to the rib area, after which an instrument would be used go through the skin, penetrate the mass and extract a tissue sample. The doctor appeared, and introduced himself and explained the procedure and what I may experience.

As he began, I was covered completely with a blue drape. The area that he was going to biopsy was exposed and the nurse cleansed it with a sterile solution. As you can imagine, the numbing of the area was the worst pain. I felt him inject the anesthesia in five different places. It stung and burned slightly, but was fairly quick-acting. I guess it was best not to be able to see what he was doing or getting ready to do. He checked the area to ensure it was, in fact, numb. He then told me I would hear a noise similar to a "spring-action" device. When that moment arrived, it sounded like the spring-loaded dart gun of my childhood, shooting plastic darts with suction cups on the ends.

The procedure took about 30 minutes from start to finish. I returned to my room around 3:30 p.m.

Todd arrived shortly thereafter, about 4:15 pm. I told him about my day and the procedures performed. Unfortunately, results from the tests would take time; results from the biopsy could take up to 48 hours.

Todd and I "dined" together in my room, and I spoke to Mom and a few others anxiously awaiting news, to bring them up to date on my condition. My nurse appeared around 7 p.m. and told me I was scheduled for a PET scan tomorrow morning at 9 a.m. I would not be able to eat or drink after midnight. If I needed to order an evening snack I should do so. So I did, we snacked, and Todd left around 8:00 p.m.

The next morning, Todd arrived at 8 a.m. sharp. He wanted to be there during the PET scan. Promptly at 9 a.m., a technician arrived and took me for my PET scan at radiology. Forty five minutes prior to the scan, I needed to drink a glucose drink. Additionally, the radiology technician injected a solution into my vein. Cancer cells thrive on sugar; by ingesting this solution, evidence of cancer would be seen on the PET scan.

The waiting area was very calm and relaxing. I was seated in a recliner with several warm blankets on me. There was soft, instrumental music playing, and the lights were dimmed. I dozed off and was awakened by the technician 45 minutes later who escorted me to the PET scan machine.

The machine was similar to a CT scan except the part you move through is about four feet wide. I took a seat on the sliding table and lay on my back. My knees were draped over a firm foam wedge, my arms were raised above my head and the technician placed a fresh, warm blanket over my arms to keep them warm.

I was told what to expect. "The sliding table will slide you into the machine and the scan will take pictures starting just below your throat on down to your thighs."

A PET scan divides the body into sections. At each section the scan take six minutes to record the data and then you slide to the next section. The scan takes a total of about 25 minutes.

The room was dimly lit. Above the machine the traditional fluorescent light covers were replaced with ones that had blue sky and clouds on them. The environment was as calm and relaxed as the waiting room.

The table began to move me into position. I was now inside the tubular machine which was just six inches above my body. As I lay there, I began to connect with my yogic breathing. I began to take long deep inhales and long exhales. My eyes closed and I dozed. The time passed quickly, and I was once again awakened by the technician at the completion of the scan. Getting into the wheelchair, I returned to my bed where Todd was waiting for me.

Todd's Take

The doctor's couldn't tell us how long Luci was going to be in the hospital. For me, the worst thing was waiting for all the results. We both just wanted this to be over. The nights at home for me were not restful. I was on the phone constantly with family and friends. When the opportunity came for sleep, I spent my time on the Internet trying to educate myself on this disease. Symptoms, diagnosis, stage evaluation and prognosis. The more I read the more worried I became. The cancer-related articles and websites were painting a pretty bleak picture. Luci's cancer still had not been "staged." I was praying that this had been caught early and it would be a relatively routine procedure.

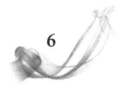

6

What's A Girl Gotta Do to Get a Drink?

*"**What happens in my room stays in my room.**"*

The waiting game was wearing on all of us. My organized self—my in control self—hated all this vagueness. I needed to know what exactly was going on. Until I knew, everything seemed surreal and unsettling.

That Tuesday, Shar was my nurse. The time was around 2 p.m. I was in the bathroom and I heard Todd conversing with her. She was asking about how he and I met; how long we've been married; if we had any children and such.

A feeling came over me suddenly that the news was not good. I exited the bathroom and asked if the results

> *"... I am really sorry to have to give you this diagnosis."*

from the scan had come back yet. Her response was, "Yes—Dr. Pinzinski would be the one to review them with us."

She left, and I said to Todd, "It's bad."

He abruptly said, "Stop it—you don't know that," but the feeling that my world was about to crumble weighed heavily upon me.

Rita arrived around 3 p.m. Shortly thereafter, Dr. Pinzinski appeared. Todd and Rita were sitting on the couch in front of the window, and I was in bed. Our conversation ended immediately as he stepped into the room.

"I reviewed the results of the PET scan and they're not good. It is ovarian cancer. There is cancer in your abdomen, in the rib area and there are two lymph nodes in the chest area that are lit up. I am really sorry to have to give you this diagnosis." I just sat there with no expression at all. I looked over toward Todd and Rita. They both began to cry.

Tears began to fill my eyes. I wanted to speak, but I was determined not to cry. I had to remain strong and in control. I then looked at Dr. Pinzinski and said, "I just need to know if I can have a glass of wine."

He replied, "You can have anything you want," and then left my room.

Rita immediately came over to my bed and got in it with me and embraced me. She said, "You cannot die, I need you." I don't really know what came over me at that Moment, but oddly, there was no emotion.

"I need the phone," pointing to the hospital phone. I picked it up and dialed "3663." I had this number memorized—room service.

A woman answered, asking, "Good afternoon, what may I get you, Ms. Berardi?"

I said, "I need a glass of wine and I would prefer white."

She said, "Pardon me?"

I repeated myself. "I said I would like to order a glass of wine; it's doctor's orders."

"I apologize, Ms. Berardi, but your doctor would need to put the order in, and this type of request would then come from the pharmacy."

Who knew you could actually get wine in a hospital?!

After I hung up the phone, Todd immediately said he would go get a bottle himself. He had noticed there was a liquor store just across the street from the hospital. He left and Rita stayed with me.

Fifteen minutes later, he returned with a bottle of Santa Margherita Pinot Grigio, one of my favorites. The bottle had already been opened and corked. The liquor store clerk had done the honors. Apparently this store gets a fair amount of business from the hospital—celebratory and otherwise.

Rita found three Styrofoam cups and Todd filled them up. I would have preferred glass, but when in Rome

… We sat together and sipped silently. It was like something you see in a movie. No one could find the right thing to say.

Shar, a few minutes later, entered the room with an immediate look of shock when she saw the open bottle of wine on my bed table. She quickly drew the curtain around my bed. "Oh my God, you can't drink that in here!"

I assured her it was fine. After all, it was "doctor's orders."

Almost immediately we fell silent to a knock at the door. We all turned our heads toward the sound. Shar stepped outside of the curtain area and opened it. Hearing her say … "Thank you," the door closed. Todd, Rita and I exchanged glances—at the same time, she pulled open the curtain and handed me a split of Beringer White Zinfandel saying it had come from the pharmacy.

I guess it was as close to white as they could find!

She then added, "I didn't even know the pharmacy had alcohol; you might as well try it."

The bottle in my hand was covered in dust. Fearing the worst, and knowing the fate of inexpensive white wine too long in the bottle, I opened it (it had a screw top) and took a swig. It was immediately obvious that there is not a big demand on the hospital pharmacy for wine. It had turned to vinegar. With a sour look as well as taste, I handed it back to Shar who dumped it down the sink. I then re-assured her, "What happens in my room stays in my room." We would keep the good bottle hidden and Todd would dispose of the evidence properly. No one would need to know. Shar just smiled and left the room.

Things started moving fast. At around 3:30 p.m. Jody, a physician's assistant, entered my room. She introduced herself and we discussed the disturbing option of having a hysterectomy. I was told Dr. Mary Jo Schmitz, a gynecological oncologist, would be in shortly. Not more than five minutes later, three more white-coated individuals appeared. Dr. Schmitz, the gynecological oncologist, Dr. Guber, a thoracic surgeon, and Kelly, who worked in genetic testing.

There I sat, along with Todd and Rita and an imposing committee of (impressively titled) physicians and (first named) assistants.

They, with my participation, proceeded to discuss my case. I voiced my biggest concern: my heart—my fear of not being able to make it through surgery. Dr. Guber suggested an epidural as the primary block and thereafter, a light, general sedation. This would help to keep the heart "dry." That was a medical term for minimizing the effort of the heart, during sedation, flushing and moving all those chemicals throughout my body. Dr. Schmitz concurred.

I felt comfortable with the discussion and the decisions—the program—that were made. I was told that both Dr. Guber and Dr. Schmitz would discuss this all with the anesthesiologist, Dr. Dale Lewis, prior to surgery.

Kelly, who works with genetic testing, then asked if I would be interested in being tested for a genetic mutation which is linked to ovarian cancer.

I agreed to the testing with the understanding that if my insurance would not cover it, I would have the option of continuing with the testing or not.

The meeting lasted about twenty minutes and then everyone left. Todd and Rita sat quietly on the couch during that time, witnessing the profound discussion of my surgical "fate." This was all so new and more than a bit overwhelming for them as well as myself. There was no viable option; I just had to go with it. Sometimes ignorance is bliss….

I immediately thought, "Oh my God, I need to tell my family." I reached for my cell phone to call my oldest brother, Frank. He was the head of the family. As far back as I could remember, there was an unwritten chain of command there. Growing up in New York of Italian descent, there were unwritten rules, and I was taught to respect them. The father is the head of the family and all things go through him first. Remember the movie *The Godfather*? An extreme example … but true.

Since my father passed away many years ago, the next in command has been his eldest son and my brother, Frank. So I scrolled through my Blackberry's address book and pressed "call." Frank answered after the first ring. With no hesitation, I blurted out, "Hi Frank, it's Lucille; the doctors just came in and I have ovarian cancer. Either you or Jerry need to tell Mom. She cannot hear this over the phone."

He replied, "I'll take care of it, Lucille."

I quickly responded, "… and Frank, make sure you tell Mom she needs to be strong and not to call me if she is going to break down and cry. I can't deal with that right now."

Again he reassured me it would be taken care of, and ended the call by saying, "I love you Lucille," to which I responded, "I love you too, Frank."

Todd's Take

When Dr. Pinsinski told us the PET results, it was like having the wind knocked out of you. I couldn't breathe, I couldn't talk. I just sat there. We like to think that when the pressure is on, we as men, can suck it up, not be emotional; be the rock for everyone to rely on. I'm sorry to say, for me, that was not the case. My eyes began to fill with tears and my throat tensed. I was in shock. In my head, I was scrolling through all the data I had read online.

Luci and Rita were in each other's arms, so I decided to walk across the street and get a bottle of wine. I couldn't wait any longer for the hospital staff to provide a glass of wine. I had no control over them or my wife's condition, but I COULD, BY GOD, get a bottle of wine for her. It didn't seem like much but I was looking for anything that I could control the outcome of—anything I could do to help my wife get through this. On the walk through the hospital corridors, I called my mother, who is a colon cancer survivor. By the time I got to the liquor store across the street from the hospital, I was relating to her Dr. Pinzinski's diagnosis. I guess the older gentleman behind the counter couldn't help overhearing my conversation. With an understanding look, he said, "I'm sorry for your news—you'll be needing this." He then handed me a small corkscrew and plastic bag to conceal my purchase.

When the trio of doctors came in later that afternoon, I was trying to keep track of everything they said. By now it had set in that this was not going to be a routine surgery. All I could do was hold Luci's hand and listen.

Mom's Take

*There were tests after tests and no answers …
This went on for two days. Finally on Tuesday, she was scheduled for a PET scan. I went to work today waiting to hear from her or Todd. No one*

called. Around 5p.m. that evening my son, Jerry, came over to my house. Right then I knew the news wasn't good. Needless to say, he said, "Mom (crying), Lucille has cancer—not good." Oh God! I felt like I had got hit by a brick. My first thought was, "No way, they must be wrong."

They kept her there and surgery was scheduled for Wednesday morning. They said it had spread to ovaries, uterus and not sure about the lungs. My little girl, why her and not me?

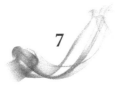

The Night Before

***I had a choice; I could either stay focused
and positive or throw in the towel and give up.***

The mystery was solved. I have ovarian cancer. At the present Moment, I could not think of a more devastating situation. Like it or not, this was my journey. I had a choice; I could either stay focused and positive or throw in the towel and give up. But, I sure as HELL was not ready to die.

Preparing for this fight, I knew it was imperative to surround myself with a network of family and friends with this same attitude, helping me stay focused and determined. I say to each of you, my readers, in your own fight: If you don't have this type of supportive network, create it! Get rid of all negatives and create the support circles that will support you and your needs.

Evening quickly settled in on us. Rita stayed with Todd and me all afternoon and into the evening. She didn't leave my side. I thought to myself, my Mom probably knows the diagnosis now and I should call her. I got out my Blackberry and dialed her number. She answered on the first ring.

"Hello!?"

I said, "Hi, Ma."

My Mom responded, "I am flying out tomorrow. What time is your surgery?" I said, "They have me scheduled for 9:30 a.m." I then asked if Aunt Lucy, my Mom's sister, who lives with my Mom, would be coming as well.

My Mom replied, "Do you want her to come; she doesn't want to burden you or upset you?"

I asked to speak her. "Hi, Aunt Lu, yes, I would like you to come. Mom is going to need your support as I go through this." She said, "Of course, whatever you think is best, Lucille. I will have Jerry book my flight right now."

When Mom was on the phone again, I quickly said, "Todd will call you back after we figure out where you'll be staying and who will be picking you up from the airport. I'll see you after surgery, I love you, Ma."

"I love you too, dear, everything will be fine, and I will see you tomorrow, Lucille." The call ended.

Meanwhile, Rita was busy researching hotels and availability of rooms near the hospital. She located a Residence Inn and Suites just minutes from the hospital with shuttle service to and from it. She made a reservation and secured all of the details. Todd then called my mother

The Night Before

back, relayed the information to her and told her Rita would be picking her and Aunt Lu up at the airport. Their flight was scheduled to arrive at 11:30 a.m.

Rita kissed me and gave me a big hug and said she would see me after surgery. She said, "I Love you, Luci, my BFF."

I responded, "I love you too, Ri," as we embraced. She gathered her things, opened the curtain, looked back one last time, smiled, blew me a kiss, and then she was gone.

Todd stayed through dinner. He gave me a kiss and said he would be back in the morning before I went into surgery.

These past three days were a whirlwind. I finally had some quiet time to just be with my thoughts by myself. I still couldn't believe what was really happening. Three days ago I was in Utah, laughing and enjoying my family. Three days ago, Todd and I were to have dinner with our good friends, Ray and Sherri. And three days ago, I came to the ER thinking I was beginning to experience the early symptoms of congestive heart failure due to my mitral valve prolapse. Now, here I was, sitting in a hospital bed the night before I was to go into surgery for a hysterectomy—and who knows what else—once they were inside of me. Three life-changing days—what was next? What would happen over the next three days?

For the first time since this whole thing occurred, it was beginning to sink in for me. I was scared! But part of me was more concerned with going under anesthesia—

the risks this would have on my heart's ability to make it through the procedure. Thankfully, I felt if I had to undergo surgery, this would be the time to do so. I contribute my strong physical and mental state of mind to my practice and to my dedication to my yoga. As I lay here in bed, I closed my eyes and once again began to reconnect with my yogic breathing. I began to pray the Rosary within my mind and drifted off to sleep.

Around 7 a.m. my cell phone rang. It was my Mom. She and Aunt Lucy had arrived at the Salt Lake City airport and were waiting for their flight to Denver. She reassured me everything would be okay and she would see me after surgery. That made me smile and I said, "Thank you, Ma, I love you."

"I love you too, dear; I will see you soon."

Hanging up, I just sat up in bed and gazed out my window. What a beautiful morning in Colorado. The sky was clear with a tint of pink and peach as the sun cast its brilliance on the Rocky Mountains. It was so peaceful and serene. As I looked outside, similar thoughts from the night before entered my mind. It still seemed surreal. In just a few hours, I would be going into surgery because I had cancer—ovarian cancer. I didn't know what to expect for recovery. I didn't know what the surgeon would find once inside, or what the steps towards recovery would involve once the surgery was over.

The Night Before

There are certain times in your life where you are not in control, and this was one of them. I must admit, being a control freak, it was hard for me to let go, but it was probably one of the greatest lessons I would come to learn from this entire experience.

> *What if Luci dies?*
> *—Todd*

Todd arrived at 8 a.m. He entered my room with a smile on his face, and said, "Hey, how are you doing." Then he came over and kissed me. I told him about my evening and updated him on my surgery status. We just sat and chatted as we waited. And there was so much that wasn't said that seemed to be said between us as we held hands, knowing the clock was ticking.

I could see the worry and concern weighing on him. I just didn't really know what to say or how to help ease his anxiety. There were so many unknowns—unknowns confronting the two of us in the upcoming months once the surgery was behind us. This man was part of me, the love of my life. Whatever the unknowns were, I silently thanked God that Todd was my partner in it.

We sat in my hospital room waiting for my turn to go to pre-op. During this time, I received several calls from friends and family wishing me well and offering me their prayers.

Suddenly there was a knock on my door and the curtain was drawn open. "Lucille?"

"Yes," I replied.

"My name is Melanie. I am going to get your surgical IV started." She came over to the right side of my bed and accessed the veins in my arm. "This one here on your forearm looks good." She wiped the area with an alcohol swab. "Ready?"

"Mother F@#$%*!!!" I exclaimed.

"Oh, I am so sorry, let me try again."

I said, "I apologize for my outburst, but we're done here. You need to get someone in here who knows what they're doing." Todd sat there in silence.

Twenty minutes later, there was another knock at the door. Two individuals entered my room—a male and a female in their mid-30s. I was puzzled by their appearance. Each of them wore a blue jumpsuit with a fluorescent yellow vest. Greg, the man, could see my confusion.

"We were told some assistance was needed to start a surgical IV. We're from the flight-for-life team. There's no vein we can't access."

I smiled and said, "I apologize now for any obscenities that may come out."

Greg laughed and replied, "If I don't hear swearing, I'm not doing my job right." I took a deep breath … and the needle was in.

At 9:30 a.m. another knock found my door.

"Lucille, they're ready for you in the OR and I'm here to escort you." The clinician was a young female about 5'9", slender build, with dark eyes and long brown hair restrained in a pony tail.

She was very friendly and invited Todd to come along with us. She told Todd to bring all of my belongings, as I would not be coming back to this room following surgery. Todd gathered up my remote office and my personal items and the three of us were off.

We arrived at the surgical floor and exited the elevator. I recall it was rather quiet in this part of the hospital.

I was greeted by the surgical prep nurse who got my IV started. Next, I saw Dr. Schmitz. She smiled and said good morning to us. She had such a warm, comforting smile, clearly meant to reassure. Next, Dr. Lewis, the anesthesiologist, appeared. He introduced himself and announced he was there to start my epidural block. I was asked to roll onto my left side and hold onto the bed rail. Todd was on that side, holding my hand. Dr. Lewis first administered an anesthetic block followed by a quick poke in the middle of my back. He completed the process by feeding a tube into my back. I remember feeling pressure, but no pain. Once he was finished, he excused himself and disappeared.

The pre-op nurse returned and told me I would need to remove my wedding band before surgery. I took off the ring and handed it to Todd. She then told Todd it was time for him to leave, and she gave us a Moment to be alone. Todd reached over and gave me a kiss. "I love you."

Tears began to fill my eyes. I responded, "I love you, too." I told him whatever Dr. Schmitz finds, I didn't want to know. I have heard enough bad news, and I did not want to hear anything else. I also asked him to make sure he tells my Mom and Aunt the same thing.

He nodded. "You got it." He gave me another kiss and squeezed my hand. He opened the curtain, looked back once more with a smile on his face, and he was gone.

Todd's Take

I knew that the distance from our house in Bailey to Swedish was much too far, especially in the case of an emergency. Her mother, Pat, needed to be close to the hospital. After talking with some of the nurses, Rita and I were able to find lodging for her and her sister, Lu. A two-bedroom condominium, five minutes from the hospital would be our home until Luci could be released. I rented it for one week, praying that the doctors' estimate on Luci's recovery would be accurate.

When Luci handed me her wedding ring, I put it on my left little finger. I told her it would be there for her when she got out of surgery and went to the OR waiting room. Alone for a few hours, the gravity of the situation began to take hold. I thought of what could happen… What are they going to find? How am I going to care for her? Will her insurance be dropped? Where is the money going to come from if I can't work?

Should I close my business? What can I sell? What are her limitations going to be? How is she going to manage getting up and down our narrow spiral staircase? How am I going to get her to her chemo treatments when the winter weather hits? Should I look for an apartment in town?

I was overwhelmed with the unknown. In the last four days, our world had crumbled. I didn't know if I could hold it together. I was scared. What if Luci dies?

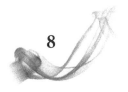

Post Surgery Recovery

"If you were to toss a cup of sugar into the air and then try to pick up each crystal individually, that's what we are dealing with. The chemotherapy will have to remove the rest."

Overall, the surgery went well. At 1:30 p.m., Dr. Schmitz came out of surgery and presented the findings to my family and friends who were anxiously awaiting the outcome. In the waiting room were Todd, Mom, Aunt Lucy, Rita, Aimee, Ray and Sherri and Ivan, one of Todd's good friends. The doctor explained that I had come through the surgery fine and my heart was doing very well.

She continued on to inform them, "It was as bad as it gets: Stage IV," explaining that the cancer had engulfed my ovaries, fallopian tubes, uterus and the entire omentum. There was also a plaque-like film on my spleen and three other areas, which she could not remove. She removed all the affected organs and areas she was able to see.

I awoke to a mostly dark room and the silhouette of a female. She introduced herself, "Lucille, I'm Rita, your nurse. You are in ICU. The surgery is over."

I remember thinking, "I made it through the surgery!" I silently said thank you to my heart. Then I began to feel pretty severe pain in my pelvic area and my back. Rita asked on a scale of 1 to 10, with 10 being the worst, how would I rate my pain? I told her it was a 9. She then told me she was going to give me Dilaudid for the pain and it should go away pretty quickly. I remember watching her as she administered the drug via a syringe into my IV line. Not five seconds after she administered the drug, I felt the effects of it. A feeling of heaviness overcame my body and my eyes drifted closed, and that's all I remember. I awoke again to severe pain in my back. It was 12:30 a.m. I called for Rita. As she entered, I was in tears from the severity of the pain. I told her she needed to call the doctor, it was unbearable. She put a call into Dr. Lewis, the anesthesiologist. "Dr. Lewis was on his way in." During the time waiting for the arrival of Dr. Lewis, Rita gave me another dose of Dilaudid.

"Lucille, it's Dr. Lewis, how are you doing?"

I told him I had excruciating pain in my lower back. He instructed Rita to assist me in turning on my left side and holding onto the bed rails. Dr Wilson removed the tube from my back and within seconds the pain was gone. What a sense of relief!

Early Thursday morning I awoke to an empty room. My first thought was, what was the time? It was 8:30 a.m. I thought, how could this be? Where is everyone; Todd, my Mom and Aunt Lu? I picked up the hospital phone and called my Mom's cell.

"Hello?"

"Where the HELL are you guys? I'm here all alone and it's 8:30 a.m."

"Okay Lucille, we're getting ready and we'll be there shortly."

"Okay, but hurry up." I was rude and demanding, but in my mind I needed to stay strong, and I was determined to get back to normal as soon I could. I needed my support team to assist in the process.

Not long after, Todd, my Mom, and Aunt Lucy appeared in my room. I was in and out of sleep throughout the entire day. Dr. Pinzinski met my mother and Aunt Lucy as he made his rounds. Later that evening I was moved from ICU to another floor.

I was assisted by my nurse and Todd to make my first attempt of getting out of bed and walking in the hallway. I couldn't believe how weak I was. It's amazing what can happen within a 24 hour period. We took it slowly and I needed both of them, one on each side of me, to accomplish this task.

A major request was to get out of this hospital gown. For the three days prior to surgery, I was adamant I was not going to be lying in bed in one of them. My attitude after surgery did not change. The solution? I knew there was a Wal-Mart just a few blocks from the hospital. I was not able to wear my yoga clothing following surgery due to the presence of a catheter, and I did not want any waist band across my abdomen over my incision site. I asked my Mom if she would go and buy me a night shirt and some slippers.

She and Todd made a Wal-Mart run. Soon they returned with a pink and blue night shirt and a pair of pink plush slippers. I can't emphasize enough how my mind-set changed once I was wearing my new threads.

On Friday morning, my younger brother, Jerry, arrived. I remember waking up and seeing him. There he was and it brought an immediate smile to my face. Jerry and I have a special bond. I was so glad and grateful that he had come, not only for me, but for Todd too. This gave Todd a diversion, and it allowed me time to be alone with Mom and Aunt Lucy.

Much of my remaining stay in the hospital was foggy. I do remember being visited by Ray and Sherri every day, and by Rita and my other very dear friend, Aimee. I was in and out of sleep most of the time and not very "social." I did remember lying in bed being concerned about the post surgical effects of carbon dioxide in my abdominal cavity and feeling the pain and discomfort associated with the trapped gas.

Because of this fear, I was determined to eat regularly and walk as much as I could.

The next challenge I faced was having a bowel movement. This was critical for many reasons but primarily to ensure my internal organs were still functioning on their own. Following this type of surgery, it is common for the organs to take three to five days to get back in sync. Having been subjected so often to so many pain medications, my body did not favor a bowel movement. It was a waiting game.

On Saturday it still had not occurred. I was now feeling the effects of the trapped gas as well as not having a bowel movement. I was very uncomfortable. I had terrible bloating and was constipated. My release from the hospital was linked to a successful bowel movement. I requested a suppository. The doctor authorized my request.

> "Woo Hoo! Luci POOPED!!"

I recalled a method I had learned at a yoga retreat on natural defecation: squatting. Modern toilets and other sitting positions, closes a portion of the colon, which can make elimination more difficult. Squatting or placing your feet on the toilet seat or on an elevated platform opens the colon, allowing better and more complete elimination.

I had done it in the past and it worked. But I knew I could not bring my feet to the toilet seat due to my incision. So I asked my Mom to find me something that I could put my feet on. She had a puzzled look on her face but didn't question my request. She came in with a rectangular trashcan. I asked her to lay it on its side so I could put my feet on it. I needed to get some elevation of my legs. It worked. I had a bowel movement! It's amazing how something as small as a bowel movement would feel like such a milestone. This news quickly spread via text messaging. "Woo Hoo! Luci POOPED!!"

Todd's Take

A nurse came out and told us Luci's surgery was complete and led Rita, Pat, Lu and myself to a small, secluded room. Dr. Schmitz would be in to talk to us in a few minutes. This was unnerving. What was she going to say? My own research had alerted me to the possibility of Stage IV and a poor prognosis. When Dr. Schmitz open the door, we all fell silent, waiting for her to speak. She politely introduced herself to Pat and Lu.

The surgery went well and Luci was going to be on her way to the ICU shortly. My worst fear was confirmed when Dr. Schmitz explained what she found. With Stage IV assured, she had removed all the cancer that she could. Unfortunately, when this cancer spreads, it spreads wildly. She explained, "If you were to toss a cup of sugar into the air and then try to pick up each crystal individually, that's what we are dealing with. The chemotherapy will have to remove the rest. I'd like to start as soon as possible." We all fell silent as tears again built up in everyone's eyes.

Dr. Schmitz asked us if we had any questions; no one responded, so she left us to ourselves. Pat and Lu silently left after a few minutes, leaving Rita and I alone. We embraced and cried together trying to compose ourselves before we went out to the main waiting room.

After about thirty minutes, Luci was ready to be rolled to the ICU. She looked so frail. I held her hand. She said, "I'm okay; I'm in pain," repeatedly as the gurney proceeded down the silent corridor. Once she was in the ICU and resting, I went to the front desk and asked if I could stay the night on the padded benches. The charge nurse told me to go home and get some sleep, I would see Luci in the morning.

Aunt Lu's Take

We waited nervously, for her to come out of surgery.

I felt very angry, sad, and I hated everyone and everything around me, when I heard of her diagnosis.

I kept thinking how could this be, our family could never be whole again without her.

9
Home Sweet Home

"Something as simple as waking up and taking a shower was no longer something I could do myself."

Recovering from surgery for those several days at Swedish, my thoughts frequently centered on home, our life there and my desire to return to it as soon as possible.

I have lived in Colorado for over 20 years and I call it home. When Todd and I met, I was living in a traditional neighborhood, in a cookie cutter style home in Parker, Colorado, a suburb of Denver, one popular for families with children. Living in Parker offers many conveniences, but I really did not appreciate the true beauty Colorado had to offer until Todd and I got together. Todd lived in a mountain town, Bailey. Bailey is located in the foothills about 45 miles southwest of Denver. At first the drive seemed long, but, over time, the drive became a meditative opportunity for me.

Our home is modest, but one that suits us perfectly. Sited on one and one third acres of wooded property, it has two stories, is cedar-sided and is literally built right into the side of a granite mountainside. Running the length of the house there is a 20 foot wide deck on which our hot tub sits.

Ponderosa pines and aspen trees surround us. Neighborhood homes are sparsely scattered about. Deer roam through our community and are tame enough to eat from your hand if one desired to do so. It was heaven.

In my austere hospital room, my thoughts returned again and again to one of our greatest joys, coming home on a Friday evening, pouring a glass of wine and soaking in our hot tub. The silence that surrounds us, the clean air that is filled with a subtle scent of pine trees, is true serenity. When will I be able to do that again?

Sunday morning the doctor came in and told me I was to be released today. Hallelujah! One thing, however, that still needed to be arranged was the delivery of oxygen to my home. Since Todd and I live at 8600 feet above sea level, the doctor was concerned with my oxygen level. I was fluctuating between 88 and 90 in the hospital at 5000 feet, so he ordered an oxygen concentrator and portable oxygen bottles to be delivered to my home.

A concern Todd had was our spiral staircase in our home. How was he going to get me upstairs? Would I even be able to get upstairs or was he going to have to transform our living room into a bedroom for me? There were many unanswered questions, and the weight on Todd was becoming evident.

At 2 p.m. I was officially released from the hospital. Getting into the vehicle was a challenge. I was so weak, and I could not stand up straight. I took one of the pillows from my room to use as a buffer across my abdomen under the seat belt. Ray and Sherri came to the hospital to help all of us get home. My Mom and I rode with Ray and Sherri. Todd drove our vehicle home with Jerry and Aunt Lucy. The ride home was about 45 minutes. Everything was going fine up until the last 15 minutes.

Suddenly, I began to get terrible pains in my stomach, which seemed to me to be trapped gas. I was concerned that I was going to shit myself. I just needed to get home as soon as possible and it took everything I had to hold it in.

Ray pulled up the driveway and I told my Mom that I needed to get out right away. Todd and Jerry were already home waiting to help me out of the vehicle which they did—first out of the car and then to the door. I was able to walk unattended, but I was not able to stand fully erect. It took every bit of energy I had in me to get myself into the house and to our bathroom.

I made it to the bathroom in time. My internal organs clearly were in turmoil from all the trauma and medication my body had been subjected to over the past week. No longer was I constipated; I now had the runs.

That little job done, I then came out of the bathroom and headed for the spiral staircase. I was determined to make it upstairs to our bedroom.

I could see the fear in his eyes as to what the future would bring.

I climbed the staircase by myself. I remember reaching the top of the stairs and looking down only to see Todd, my Mom, Aunt Lu, Jerry, Ray and Sherri just standing at the bottom of the stairs in silence and amazement. I entered our bedroom and got into bed ... all by myself.

Todd entered shortly thereafter to make sure I was comfortable and if I needed anything. I said "No, I'm just gonna take a nap now." He kissed me on the forehead, smiled and closed the door behind him. Ray and Sherri went home.

The oxygen company arrived around 4 p.m. with my oxygen concentrator and my portable units. The representative went over all the procedures and instructions with Todd. As a precautionary measure, I began full-time oxygen usage shortly thereafter.

Evening quickly set in. I spent the evening upstairs. Sherri and Ray brought dinner to us this evening. A baked ham, mashed potatoes, green beans, rolls and a carrot Jell-O mold. Mom prepared a plate and Todd brought it up to me on a bed tray. My appetite was returning. So was my pain—shortly thereafter, I took another Vicodin and drifted off to sleep.

Waking up in my own bed seemed like such a milestone for me. Just one week ago I was told I had cancer, and the thought did enter my mind, would I ever see my home again? The sun filled our bedroom and I awoke with Todd at my side. I must say, all in all, I really did not have much pain from the surgery itself. The incision was healing very nicely. The pain I was still experiencing was that of trapped gas in my abdomen. Mom brought me some toast and hot tea. I had no strength or energy to do anything but lay in bed. I remained in my bedroom throughout the day. I spent much of it visiting with my brother Jerry. I could see the fear in his eyes as to what the future would bring. He provided me a great deal of comfort and I just held on to every minute we had together, for I knew his visit was coming to an end. The following morning, Todd drove Jerry to the airport. Another beautiful, sunny fall morning began to unfold.

I hated feeling like a prisoner in my own bedroom. Over the past week, I had lost ten pounds. Something as simple as waking up and taking a shower was no longer something I could do by myself. I truly did not have the strength to take a shower. I so wanted to get some normalcy back into my life. I asked Todd if he could help me. I just knew if I could wash my hair and my body, I would feel better. Todd said yes, but he had to prepare the bathroom and left the room.

He returned about ten minutes later and said the bathroom was now ready. Helping me out of our bed, he walked me to the bathroom where—surprise—there in the bathtub was a shower chair. Ray had brought it over for me to use.

Earlier this year Ray had hip surgery and found this chair to be very useful. Todd had also replaced the shower head with a hand-held massaging unit. He helped me undress and get seated on the chair; then he handed me the massaging unit and turned the water on. I drew the curtain and Todd stepped outside of the bathroom.

It felt wonderful to take a shower, but I couldn't believe how exhausted I was afterwards. For the first time I actually had time with myself and saw how thin and frail I really was.

I called for Todd when I was done and he helped me out of the shower, and, with his help, I got dressed. He then walked me back to our bedroom where my mother was busy changing the bedding and getting a load of laundry ready. I asked him to get my hair dryer and to bring in the shower chair for me to sit on.

My mother came over and told me to sit down and rest and she would dry my hair for me. Todd returned with the chair, hair dryer and brush and handed them to her. He asked if I needed him to help with anything else. I just smiled and said, "No I'm fine. Mom and I can handle this; thank you, babe." I was determined to dry my own hair.

Mom patiently sat on the side of the bed watching me. It's amazing what we take for granted. I knew I had a lot of hair but I never noticed before how long and thick it really was until this morning when I was drying and drying it. It seemed forever; I could no longer continue. My arms became very tired and weak. She could see the effort it was taking, came over with a gentle touch and, smiling at me, took the hair dryer and finished what I had started. This was all I was going to accomplish today. I returned to my bed and just read for a while. Mom left the room without saying a word. She knew I needed some time alone.

My discomfort worsened as I began to experience the residual effects of the trapped gas in my shoulder. As much as I hated taking pain medication, I continued to take it to help with the discomfort at night. I was desperate to find some remedies to help with the trapped gas. I sat in my bed with my laptop, in search of answers on the Internet. I happened upon one woman's blog with a possible solution; she recommended walking and rocking in a chair to help release the gas.

I clearly wasn't up to taking a walk outside at this point, but I thought I could manage to walk back and forth on the deck off of our bedroom. I called to my Mom and asked her to help me. I never realized how restricted one must feel when they are dependent on oxygen. I was given a 100 foot hose to allow me to move throughout our home, but I often forgot I was connected by that tube to the oxygen bottle. More than once, I got tangled up or had the tube pulled from my face.

When I was ready to walk, Mom and I ventured outside through the master bedroom onto the deck. The sun was shining brightly and, I must say, it felt wonderful on my face.

I did four laps back and forth on the deck in hopes of dismissing some of the gas. It seemed to help a bit, but there was clearly still a problem. When I returned to the bedroom, I asked her to lay my yoga mat out for me. On it I bent down and brought myself into a devotional pose. Again, it was another attempt to assist the gas to leave my body. And it felt good on so many levels.

This was the first time since before my diagnosis that I was able to come to my mat and reconnect with my inner self. A feeling of peace and calm overcame me. I just lay there breathing. I don't know how long I was there, but when I came up out of the pose, I was the only one in my room. And I felt better.

Later that evening I ventured downstairs for the first time, Todd stood at the bottom of the spiral stairs, I'm sure just in case he needed to respond quickly if I took a tumble or couldn't make it.

All went well. I came down by myself and sat in my recliner … a successful descent.

Mom's Take

My son booked a flight for me and my sister for the following morning to Colorado. When we got there, Lucille was still in surgery. We waited and waited. It seemed no one was coming to tell us her condition. Finally her surgeon came out and had a consultation with all of us. She said, "I am so sorry, Luci is full of cancer, Stage IV, but I am very hopeful.

I wanted to scream. This can't be! I thought the worst."

The road ahead we knew would be so rocky but we had to put our feelings aside and think of her and Todd. I couldn't stay there continuously and when I was at home—not knowing what she was going through—was the worst for me.

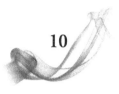

The Port

"Okay Luci, you are going to feel a poke and a burning sensation." I closed my eyes and took a deep breath.

I now have been home for five days. Today, I was scheduled for my one week, postoperative appointment with Dr. Schmitz, and I was also scheduled to have my port placed for my upcoming chemo treatment. A port is a cylinder with a hollow space inside that is sealed by a soft top. It connects to a small, flexible tube called a catheter. A special needle is used to access the port. This device provides an easy way to receive chemotherapy and have blood samples withdrawn. Additionally, the port helps to reduce the fear factor of having to receive multiple needle "sticks." In most cases, only one "stick" is needed.

My bowels seemed to be getting a little better, but what I feared was beginning to occur. Even though the pain and presence of the trapped gas seemed to have dissipated, I was now developing a hemorrhoid.

What could possibly happen next? I just knew this was going to happen; I had experienced the same type of recovery during a previous abdominal surgery when I had a fibroid removed laproscopically five years ago. It has only been ten days since my surgery and I still was not feeling great. I increased the stool softener to twice a day in hopes of minimizing the discomfort and presence of the hemorrhoid.

Mom, Aunt Lucy, Todd and I left home around 9 a.m. enroute to the hospital 45 minutes away, for my appointments. What once seemed to be done so effortlessly and without thought now became a step-by-step process. Getting in and out of our SUV took assistance from Todd and my Mom. While riding, due to the site of my incision and the lap belt, I still needed to have a pillow placed across my abdomen.

During the drive to the hospital a realization set in. A song came on the radio, *Teenage Dream* by Katy Perry. I have heard this song many times before, but today the words resonated with me … For me, something about the lyrics to this song, seemed to summarize what Todd and I shared together. I began moving to the beat as I sat in the front seat. As I listened to the song today, my eyes began to fill with tears as she sang the verse, "I finally found my missing puzzle piece, I'm complete." Todd and I had only been brought together such a short time ago, and for a moment I was scared the cancer may take this away from me.

When we arrived at the hospital, Todd quickly came around to my side of the car to help me out. I opened the door and was ready to hop out, but to my chagrin, I again needed his assistance to get out of the car. Tears began to fill my eyes. For the first time since my diagnosis, I realized how sick I really was. Even though mentally I was the same person from a week ago, my physical self was very, very ill. I still needed considerable assistance for the most ordinary things. With this realization weighing me down, the four of us walked to the elevator and proceeded to the second floor.

My postoperative visit went well. I was healing within normal limits. My weight was 104 pounds, down a remarkable 14 pounds from just one week ago. I was given a tour of the office and was shown the chemo room. I was shocked to see how full it was, with all ten recliner chairs occupied. This was an eye opening experience for me. I was scheduled for next Thursday, October 28th, at 8:00 a.m., for my first chemotherapy appointment.

Next, we headed across the pedestrian walkway to the outpatient surgery. I checked in and was prepped for my surgical procedure. Mom and Aunt Lucy had to wait in the recovery waiting room but Todd remained until they were ready for me. We just waited and watched TV for

"Are you doing okay? We are just about ready to begin."

about an hour. Then there was a knock on the wall, the curtain opened and a nurse appeared. She introduced herself and told us the doctor was ready for me. Todd now needed to go to the waiting room. The procedure would take about 20 minutes, and she would come and get him when they were finished. Todd kissed me, and she wheeled me away.

As with all operating rooms, it was cold and white and I was surrounded by a lot of big machines. The surgeon came in, introduced himself and reviewed the procedure with me. Echoing the nurse, he said it would take about 20 minutes. To begin, the anesthesiologist would give a small dose of fetinol to place me in a twilight sleep. He would then numb the area with lidocaine, make an incision to place the port in my upper right chest area just below my clavical and then make another incision to feed the tube from the port into an artery in my neck.

I explained to the surgeon my concern with anesthesia and my mitral valve prolapse; I asked him if this procedure could be done without being put under sedation. He said yes, the recovery would, in fact, be quicker due to not having the anesthesia. He warned me, however, that the experience would be more pleasant if I was under anesthesia, but it could be tolerated without sedation. The only other concern he had was if I was claustrophobic. Curious as to why, but not asking, I told him I did not have any problems with that. Agreeing to perform the procedure under local anesthetic, he asked the nurses attending, to get me prepped for the procedure and left the room.

They quickly moved about to get the room ready. I was transferred to the surgical table and covered with two warm blankets. A blue drape was then placed over my entire body including my head. Now I knew why he was concerned if I had any issues with being in closed places. The nurse informed me the surgeon would cut a hole in the drape just over the surgical site and the drape would remain covering the rest of my body during the procedure.

The surgeon returned and placed his hand on my right shoulder. "Are you doing okay; we are just about ready to begin."

I responded, "Yes," and told him I would be going to my yogic place. He need not be alarmed by my deep breathing.

He said, "Okay, Luci, you are going to feel a poke and a burning sensation." I closed my eyes and took a deep breath.

Prior to my diagnosis, I would get worked up at the sight of a needle. I guess after being stuck so many times over the past week, I clearly had learned to deal with it. Just one of the many lessons I would come to learn from this life-changing experience.

The procedure went well. Not having the sedation gave me a sense of being in control, and by this time, knowing how much my body had already been through; I knew what was coming in the very near future.

I have to say, it really wasn't that bad. The only thing I would caution one about is the sensation during the placement of the port. Once the area was numbed, however, I felt no pain at all. I only felt the two initial injections, one at the site where the port was placed and one at the site where the tube was fed into my artery.

To draw on a real-life, food-preparation analogy, the procedure itself would best be compared to making stuffed pork chops. You need to make a pocket into a thick raw pork chop by sawing and cutting though the fibers of the meat. In this case, the pork chop was the flesh—the tissues—of my own body!

Since I didn't have sedation, I was reunited with Todd, my Mom and Aunt Lucy right away, without having to be in recovery. I told them that I was very hungry. Aunt Lucy got right on it and found my nurse. Another benefit of not having sedation was being able to order food to satisfy my hunger. I had to remain in post op for two hours following the procedure, however, before I could be released.

Aunt Lu's Take

I was to stay with her now, after the port, during her first chemo treatments which were to follow ... I prayed that she wouldn't have any bad reactions.

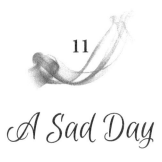

11

A Sad Day

*"I love you Lucille; everything will be okay.
I will be back soon."*

Following my release from the hospital, Todd was concerned to leave me alone at home. He spoke with our family and coordinated everyone's schedule to ensure someone would be with me at all times during my chemotherapy. Aunt Lucy was first up. My aunt deserves more credit than she is often given. She has suffered from Obsessive Compulsive Disorder (OCD) for most of her life, yet when there is any type of crisis, she is right on it and is in total control of the situation. It's as if the OCD is gone.

Mom was flying back to Utah this afternoon and this was a very tough day for me. She came up to my room and began to cry. Giving me a big hug and a kiss, she said,

"I love you Lucille; everything will be okay. I will be back soon."

I too began to cry and said, "I love you too, Mom." Prior to her departure, she prepared several meals and placed them in the freezer for us to eat in the coming days. Todd drove her to the airport and Aunt Lucy and I stayed home. Today sucked. I stayed in my room for the remainder of the day.

Saturday was a better day. Ray and Sherri came down today to visit me and stayed for about an hour. I did notice that I was beginning to cough a little, though, when I was lying down. I didn't want to alarm anyone so I kept it to myself. I went to bed early this evening.

Around 1 a.m. Sunday morning, I woke up with the same sensation of heaviness in my chest and difficulty breathing deeply. I woke Todd up and told him what I was experiencing and thought we should go to the hospital. I went into the guest room to wake up Aunt Lucy. I told her I was having trouble breathing and I thought it would be best to go the hospital. She jumped right up and said, "Okay, don't worry, I'm coming with you; just give me five minutes to get dressed."

I returned to my room and packed an overnight bag; I had a feeling I would not be coming home right away. Todd quickly gathered the dogs, put them into their kennel in the garage and started our SUV to get it warmed up. The three of us were out the door within 30 minutes. What a team I had!

A Sad Day

Once again, we were headed to the ER on a Sunday. When we arrived, I was admitted right away due to my history and my current symptoms. Fluid was beginning to build in my right pleural sac. The treating physician discussed doing another pleuradesis to remove the fluid but felt it might be best to wait until morning to visit with the pulmonologist. I agreed; I was not looking forward to another draining procedure right now.

My first thought was disappointment, but I quickly shifted my mind-set: Oh well, so be it."

I was admitted to the hospital and was brought to my room within an hour of my arrival to the ER. Aunt Lucy told Todd she would stay with me and encouraged him to go home. I too told Todd I would be fine here. There was no reason for him to stay. He should go home and get some sleep and tend to the dogs. I would call him later this morning. Todd agreed and departed.

The room was on the post-natal floor and was quite large. There was a recliner which opened to a twin-sized bed. Aunt Lucy made sure I was comfortable and then settled into the recliner. Around 7 a.m., she and I were awakened by Dr. Jennifer Wink, the pulmonologist. She listened to my lungs and told me she had spoken with Dr. Hoeffer, the thoracic surgeon, who would be in shortly to discuss my options. Dr. Wink explained to me what was occurring.

The presence of the tumor in the rib area is preventing my body's natural ability to resorb fluid. The fluid is being trapped in the pleural sac, which surrounds the lung. I was given a handout which explained the Pleuradesis procedure. She seemed optimistic, and would be back later this morning after my visit with Dr. Hoeffer.

About an hour later, he arrived. He was an associate of Dr. Guber, the surgeon who I had met with the afternoon before my hysterectomy. Dr. Guber was instrumental in coordinating with Dr. Schmitz and the anesthesiologist, Dr. Lewis, on how to proceed with my mitral valve prolapse. I did ask where Dr. Guber was, since I already had a (limited) relationship with him. Unfortunately, he was off for a few days hunting.

My first thought was disappointment, but I quickly shifted my mind-set: Oh well, so be it. I am sure he is as capable as Dr. Guber. After all, he was an associate, and he had access to Dr. Guber's prior recommendations. Dr. Hoeffer began to review the Pleurodesis procedure. I had been totally open to the recommended surgical procedures and felt completely comfortable with the care I had received up to that point.

In my mind, my first and foremost concern was my heart and how a procedure would affect it and ultimately, affect my ability to come through the procedure.

When Dr. Hoeffer asked me if I had any questions, I replied,

> Well, yes I do. I have a mitral valve prolapse with severe regurgitation. At some point after I get through all of this, I am going to need a valve repair. Will this affect my ability to be a candidate for minimally invasive surgery?

He answered,
> That is a very good question, and yes it would affect your ability to potentially have minimally invasive surgery. You would not be able to have that type of procedure done.

The Pleurodesis procedure is designed to seal the membranes around the lungs to prevent fluid build-up. This procedure is accomplished by inserting a talc-like substance. Once the substance is in place, a surgeon will no longer be able to penetrate that seal between the ribs, which is needed to perform a valve repair by entering through the ribs. The only option would be to cut through the complete rib cage, which would be major surgery.

"Well, that made this decision easy. I'm not doing the Pleurodesis with talc. What other options do I have?"

He said a drainage tube could be inserted into the rib area into the pleural sac. I would have an external tube extending out of my rib which would provide a "manual" way to drain the fluid. Again, this made my decision very easy.

I have known for years, that some day in the future I would need to have heart surgery, and my hope has always been and still remains to have my valve repaired without having to saw through my rib cage. All I was concerned about was long-term. After all this cancer stuff is over, I would need heart surgery, and I was not about to throw away my chance at minimally invasive surgery to repair my heart valve. I was open to placing the drainage tube, but not the Pleurodesis procedure with the talc.

He said to me, "I think that is a wise choice; I happen to agree with you completely." I was told there was a video which I would be required to watch before I could sign the consent form. Saying he would see me tomorrow morning to do the procedure, he left my room.

Todd showed up at 8:30 a.m. Shortly after, Ray and Sherri arrived too. I got them caught up on what had taken place this morning. My nurse came in to let me know she had set up the video for the Pleurex Drainage Tube for me to watch. This obviously would not have been my first choice of video, nor venue, but at least I had wonderful company. All that was missing was the popcorn!

Aunt Lucy, Todd, Ray, Sherri and I all proceeded down the hallway into a nurse's station. The video was fed through the Internet. I was seated in front of the computer and everyone else gathered around me. Lasting 20 minutes, the video showed how the tube is inserted under local anesthesia; how to drain the fluid using a vacuumed bottle; and how to care for the tube. In addition, there were testimonials from other patients who had undergone the procedure and their positive comments about the procedure and how the Pleurix drainage tube had helped them. I have to admit, it didn't seem too bad. So that was that; this time tomorrow I would have a drainage tube.

Ray and Sherri encouraged Aunt Lucy to go with them to the cafeteria to get something to eat. We were so caught up with everything going on, she hadn't had anything to eat since last night. The four of them left, giving Todd and I a chance to be alone. I could see the worry in his eyes, but I didn't know what to say or do. We just sat together in my bed and watched TV.

Todd's Take

One thing that Luci and I hold dear, are our relationships with our parents and siblings. When the diagnosis was clear and we knew what to expect in coming months, I reached out to my parents. I was hesitant at first but I knew I was in over my head. I was able to coordinate times that we could have family members (hers and mine) come and stay with Luci. This way, I could keep my business running and maintain some income. No one balked at my request to stay with us for a week or more. When you hear, "What can I do to help?" don't be afraid to ask.

Not everyone was comfortable driving the mountain roads so when Luci was scheduled for chemotherapy, I made adjustments on my job schedule to accommodate her appointments. Every week had to be accounted for. I wanted someone to be with Luci at all times. Trips to DIA were made nearly twice a week to pick-up or drop off someone. During those hours, Ray and Sherri were available in case something should arise.

It's funny how something as simple as how to place the flatware in a dishwasher can throw you off. We all have our own way of doing daily chores. Though frustrating at times, I knew that I could not let trivial matters detract us from the goal of Luci's eventual triumph. All in all, I can say that our family and friend support system was just as important as the chemotherapy was to Luci's recovery.

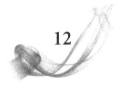

12

Rapunzel, Let Go Of Your Beautiful Hair

"The loss of my hair was one of the most emotional crosses I had to bear ..."

I don't know about other people's reaction to chemotherapy, but I can tell you mine. I've been given a lot of information over the past week and a half, most of which was not good. But the reality of losing my hair was truly a challenge. Yes, it's just hair, and it will grow back ... but ...

This is far less invasive than major surgery, an insertion of a tube or being pumped full of poison, all of which I have undergone, or am about to, yet it still was more fearful and scary to me than the above-mentioned. It's a kind of painless "amputation" of an appendage.

We are surrounded by hair in our lives; it is everywhere we look, visually and as a symbol. It is associated with beauty, confidence, and sexuality. Is it true or right?… Yes and no, but it still exists. We are told, beauty comes from within. Yeah, we've all heard it. I am here to tell you, when you're the one faced with losing your hair, that familiar saying doesn't help the situation. The loss of my hair was one of the most emotional crosses I had to bear … but the traumatic lessons I later learned far exceeded that initial trauma.

I'm not proud to admit it, but I loved my hair. I would even go so far as to say I was more than a bit obsessive about my hair. I have not had many hair dressers. When I was able to make my own decision as to my hair styles, I began seeing a guy named John in Utah. I saw him for years. Even after I moved to Colorado with Continental Airlines, I would fly back to Utah to see John for anything that revolved around my hair. John was my hair partner for 12 years, until one day he just vanished. No one knew what happened to him—where he went.

This forced me to find someone new. I found a woman in Colorado who I saw three times, but at the last visit she cut my hair shorter than I asked, and she was done. I was then introduced to Aimee's hairdresser, John. Yes, another John. She went with me so I could meet him … okay, so I could *interview* him. I really liked him. And, guess what, I have been seeing John for ten years!

Reflecting back, I had an aberration. Ever since I was a little girl, I always had long, thick, dark hair. I would attribute this to my father. He loved my long hair and would never let my Mom cut it. He had always said if I wanted to cut my hair he would be fine with my choice, but no one else would make that choice for me. One time my Mom decided to cut bangs. This did not go over very well, and needless to say, she did not do that again. Even when I was an adult, his favorite picture of me was when I was six years old with my long locks. This was the picture he had on his desk until the day he died.

When I knew I was going to lose my hair, I knew I had to have a plan. So I called Aimee and started crying to her about losing my hair. I told her there was no way I could bear to lose my long locks and that I needed to see if John would come to my house to cut my hair. I did not care about the cost I just needed this done before I started chemotherapy next week. Aimee replied, "I'm on it; don't worry about it. I will call John right now." Everything was set. On Sunday, Aimee would pick John up and drive him to my house. The only problem was the unforeseen visit to the hospital in the early hours of Sunday morning.

As Todd and I were lying in my bed watching TV, it dawned on me. I jumped up and said, "Oh My God, Aimee's supposed to bring John to our house this morning to cut my hair." I grabbed my phone and called Aimee. I told her what had happened and asked her if she could get in touch with John. About an hour later, Aimee and

Chris entered my room. I could tell by Chris' demeanor if it weren't to give his friend Todd, moral support, he'd rather be elsewhere. I looked at her and asked, "Is John on his way?"

> *Just make a ponytail and cut it!!*

She said, "There's a slight problem; he already had plans for the afternoon. John was planning on being home by 3 p.m." What???!!!, coming to the hospital is actually closer than driving all the way to Bailey. We're talking one-hour, tops.

"What could be so important?" She was hesitant; I could tell she didn't want to tell me. I persisted.

"He has a Bronco's party to go to." I was shocked. I asked her to call him again and tell him how important this was and that I was going to have another surgical procedure tomorrow and I had no idea how I would be feeling after the procedure.

Chemotherapy was set for Thursday and I needed to have this done now. She called him back. As she was talking to him, she was repeating his responses to me. At one point he told Aimee, "Just make a ponytail at the nape of the neck and cut it."

JUST MAKE A PONYTAIL AND CUT IT!! I couldn't believe what I was hearing. I took the phone from Aimee.

"Hi, John, it's Luci. I am having another surgical procedure tomorrow. I don't know what I am going to feel like afterwards. This would really mean a lot to me. If you left right now, you'd be back home in an hour."

John, to his credit, did finally agree. I handed the phone to Aimee and she told him to call her when he got to the hospital and someone would come down to meet him.

Approximately 30 minutes later, Aimee's phone rang and the room when silent. "Okay, Todd and Chris will be right down." With all the stress of the last few weeks, I know Todd was ready to blow up; I just hoped it wouldn't be with John today.

Meanwhile, Aunt Lucy had already been in contact with my nurse. She got four disposable mattress/bed pads and arranged them on the floor and placed the vanity chair in the center. A quick knock at the door was heard and there appeared Todd and John, and Chris following behind. I got up and greeted him. "Thank you John, for coming."

I sat down in the chair and tears began to fill my eyes. John covered me with a cloak and sprayed down my hair. He brushed it and gathered it into a ponytail. He placed his hand on my shoulder and said "Are you ready?" I just nodded. It took three cuts through the tail to completely sever through my hair. I just sobbed.

Everyone's eyes were filled with tears. The emotion in the room was intense. I think the urgency and importance of my request had truly set in for John. He added some shape to my new shoulder-length hairdo. Then he gave me a big hug and was gone.

The heartache I was experiencing within was twofold, loss of my beautiful hair and loss of a friend. Only later would I gain an understanding and forgiveness of John's initial reluctance to come to the hospital.

Todd's Take

I have shaved my head every March for St. Baldrick's since before Luci and I got together. For me it is just hair. For Luci, her hair was her identity. I knew this would be the most difficult hurdle for her to overcome. We had discussed donating her hair to "Locks of Love," which sounded like a good idea. In reality, she was not ready to cut the required 12" for a donation. With everything else, it was too much to part with.

When we went to the ER on Sunday morning, my nerves were shot. When I heard that John, whom I had never met, was not able to come to the hospital due to a Bronco game, I was confused. He had previously agreed to drive fifty miles to Bailey ... this was the only stylist she had allowed cut her hair for the past ten years. He had to know

this was not just a client, and Luci was in the hospital, fighting for her life. When I first heard of the apprehension, I thought he had tickets to the game. Understandably, it was a Bronco/Raider game, surely he could stop in after the game.
As the conversation deepened, I realized he was watching the game on TV. I looked at Chris and mumbled, "Have you ever heard of a DVR? ASSHOLE."

While Aimee and Luci implored John to come to the hospital, Chris and I offered to pick him up if he was concerned about drinking and driving. When he declined that offer, Chris and I pondered the possibility of abduction. The next step was to get his address and kidnap John, the hairstylist!

To his credit, John eventually relented and agreed to come to the hospital. When Luci told him Chris and I would meet him at the ER entrance, I could not wait. On the way down, Chris mentioned that it might not be in Luci's best interest to piss this guy off. So be it. I introduced myself and thanked John for making the trip.

The gravity of the situation hit him when he walked into the room and saw how thin and frail Luci had become. He asked her what she'd like to do. He then carefully cut her ponytail and styled her now shoulder length hair as everyone in the room tearfully watched. When it was done, he gathered his tools, gave her a hug and quietly left. The Denver Broncos lost to the Oakland Raiders that Sunday.

Aunt Lu's Take

My niece was trying to spare herself some pain. So she had her hair dresser come to the hospital to cut her long hair. Because she was told it would fall out completely. We waited for him to come for hours and finally he cut her hair and the look on her face as she saw her beautiful hair falling on the floor was heartbreaking.

Her hair dresser is very fortunate I or others didn't punch him because he showed no compassion for her distress and pain.

Who did he think he was—someone very great and important? Well, that is crap.

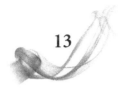

13

The Pleuradesis

"I'm tough; hell, I just went through major surgery, the placement of a port and had to have all my beautiful hair cut off. This was nothing."

Monday morning came quickly. Todd and I had discussed the evening before the surgery and his being there. I insisted that it wasn't necessary for him to be there before I went in, as Aunt Lucy would be with me and I would be fine. I was expecting a similar time line to that of the placement of my port. I told him I would rather he come to the hospital later in the day after the procedure. About 9:30 a.m., Ray and Sherri showed up. Whenever they came to see me they had big smiles on their faces. Their cheerfulness always lifted my spirits. They wanted to come to see me and to sit with Aunt Lu during the procedure—I was really happy to see them and I knew that Aunt Lu would enjoy their company.

About 10 a.m., a technician entered my room and said they were ready for me in the OR. Aunt Lucy came over to the bed, gave me a kiss and said, "Everything will be fine; I will be waiting here for you." Ray and Sherri too gave me a hug and kiss and wished me well. The clinician removed my oxygen and reconnected me to a portable unit which he laid by my side. He then released the bed brake and off we went.

I was brought to a pre-op room where the surgical nurses took my vitals. I told the nurse I did not want to be sedated due to my heart condition; I would prefer to have a local block. I thought this could not be any worse than the port, and there was the fact that there would not be any post-surgical recovery. I could get back to my room immediately and not be all drugged up. The control side of me wanted to be aware of what was going on.

"I'm tough, hell; I just went through major surgery, the placement of a port and had to have all my beautiful hair cut off. This was nothing."

Within 30 minutes, my nurse told me that the doctor's ready. Wheeling me to the operating room, I found the room similar to when I had my port placed—very cold, white and full of large lights and machinery.

Dr. Hoeffer entered and said, "Good morning, Lucille, how are you doing?"

I responded, "I'm feeling fine. How long should this procedure take?"

"About 20 minutes." He then confirmed my request not to have any sedation.

I said "Yes, I would like to do this with just a local block."

"No problem, the procedure may actually be even less than 20 minutes. Okay then, let's begin."

Again, my body was covered with a blue sterile drape. A hole was made where the surgery was to be performed and I could feel my rib area being cleansed by a cold solution. Dr. Hoeffer then said, "You will feel a poke and a stinging sensation."

Two more injections followed. I just brought myself to my yogic place. My eyes were closed and I was breathing slow and deep. After those two injections, I knew that there were more injections being done but all I felt was pressure—I felt no pain.

Dr. Hoeffer then said, "You will feel another stinging sensation," as he numbed the area on my side. This was apparently the place where he would feed the tube into the rib.

He was right—the procedure itself took about 15 minutes. As he finished up, he said it went well and that his office would be contacting me for a follow-up visit in about 10 days.

When Dr. Hoeffer left the room, I was transferred from the surgical table to my hospital bed. A technician rolled me back to my room where I was greeted by Aunt Lucy, Ray and Sherri. Telling them that the procedure went well, my hunger overtook me. All I could think about was ordering some food.

My hospital room was like a revolving door. Todd arrived around 2 p.m. and Ray and Sherri left, giving me another big hug and kiss, saying that they would see me either tomorrow or Wednesday.

Todd and I spent the afternoon just catching up—he about his day and I telling him about the procedure that I had gone through. While we chatted, Aunt Lucy took advantage of this time to go down to the cafeteria to get something to eat. Todd looked really, really tired I could see the effects of this whole ordeal intensifying for him. He stayed until about 6:30 p.m. and then got up to go home. I told him not to worry about tomorrow because Rita would be here in the morning to pick Aunt Lu and me up and would bring us home.

"Have a restful night. I'll see you tomorrow afternoon back home," I said, giving him a good night hug and a kiss.

The next day, Rita arrived around 11 a.m. I was in the bathroom getting ready as the discharge nurse entered my room. Rita was sitting on my bed talking with Aunt Lucy and the nurse thought she was me. "You look wonderful," she said.

"Uh, thank you, but I'm not the patient, she's in the bathroom."

At that Moment, I came out of the bathroom. You could see by the look on the nurse's face, she was quite embarrassed. She quickly reviewed post-operative instructions with me and left the room. The three of us burst out in laughter.

As I waited for the finalization of my release, I placed an order for some lunch. At one o'clock, I was free to go.

On the way home, I asked Rita if we could stop by a wig shop that was in partnership with the American Cancer Society. She said "Absolutely!" About 20 minutes later, we arrived at Exempla St. Luke's Hospital where Hope's Closet Gift Shop was located. The three of us were the only ones in the gift shop at the time. The volunteer, Cynthia, was so friendly. I shared with her my brief story and asked her if she had any wigs that I could try on.

She escorted us into a private room where sat a vanity with several mirrors surrounding it. There were a few wigs that we were able to look at and try on. As I put the first wig on, tears began fill my eyes. Even though I knew it was inevitable I was going to lose my hair, I don't think it had really sunk in, until this very Moment. Nothing I saw worked, making me feel even worse; tears spilled over. Then, out of the corner of my eye, two knitted caps caught my attention. Cynthia noticed and suggested another. A jersey type cap. She shared that many women find a cap helpful to sleep with. Not only does it keep the strands of hair from getting all over the pillow, it helps to reduce friction on your head and helps to retain body heat. This was all useful information to me—I hadn't thought about any of those things. I was very grateful to have stopped in there today.

Aunt Lucy, Rita, and I arrived back home around 4 p.m. Although I had only been away two days, it was a wonderful feeling to once again be back home. In my mind, just being able to return home was such a huge accomplishment. Over these past three weeks, I did have periods of hesitation as to whether or not I would actually return home again. I could also sense a sigh of relief from Aunt Lucy as well. Being back gave us all a much welcomed chance for some down-time before Thursday. Chemo day.

> *Take advantage of the many resources available to you through the American Cancer Society, like Hope's Chest.*

Todd and I took advantage of the evening to share our day with one another. I was feeling fairly good and he seemed to be more rested. He told me he had seen Dawn, our acupuncturist, for his routine visit. She was very concerned with my progress and had been in contact with him since my initial diagnosis. During his visit, she shared with him her recommendation for me to start taking an herbal supplement during chemotherapy. This supplement has been known to help minimize the side effects of chemotherapy, by tonifying qi and harmonizing the stomach. The two most fundamental forms of qi are Yin-qi and Yang-qi—the primordial feminine and masculine energies. The fundamental insight of Chinese Medicine is that free-flowing qi results in health; while stagnant or imbalanced qi leads to disease. The herbal supplement she recommended, CR Support, is manufactured by Evergreen Herbs of California. Dawn had printed out the supplement information and suggested I show it to my oncologist to get her approval. I have always been open to alternative therapies and that was the case now even more than ever. What could I possibly lose? Not a thing, but I had everything to gain. CR support would be added to my shopping list.

Aunt Lu's Take

> … She landed back in the hospital because her lungs filled with fluid again. This was a very upsetting time. She had a tube put in her side to drain it … This was hard for us to see, because it was painful for her.

14

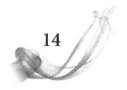

The Wall of Intention

I was determined to stay as positive as I could, especially now, since I would soon be starting chemo and had no idea what to expect.

The past two weeks had been unpredictable at best. During that trying time, I was beginning to get to know a whole new me. Someone who was very organized and in control was now "going with the flow" and, more times than not, with the turmoil, making decisions on the fly. Right now, it's been three weeks since my initial surgery. Todd was at work, Aunt Lucy was resting and I was really trying to savor this Moment of calmness and peace.

I finally had the energy and the time to attend to the mound of mail that had been piling up on the kitchen table. I gathered it up and sat on our couch where the sun

The Wall of Intention

was shining though the wall of picture windows in our living room. How I loved this spot—another glorious morning "on the mountain." Rafferty had decided to assist me in the task. He just helped himself to the other end of the couch and then rested his head on my lap. Very helpful. This was nice.

As I began to sort through the mail, I could not believe how many cards there were for me … Cards from family members, friends, co-workers, and my yoga students, all sending me their well wishes toward a speedy recovery. Tears began to fill my eyes. I never really thought about how many people my life had touched. I felt so lucky to be surrounded by their genuine prayers and intentions.

"Perfect. This is just perfect."

Later that evening, as soon as Todd came home, he came upstairs to check on me. When he entered our bedroom, there, neatly displayed across our dressers and our cedar chest, were all the get-well cards. I could see that he was as surprised as I was. I smiled and said, "I know, can you believe it?' I told him I needed to have these cards in our bedroom. I wanted to have a constant reminder of all the love and prayers being sent to me, and I wanted these cards to be the first thing I saw every morning and the last thing I saw before going to sleep.

He said, "I know exactly what to do," and he was gone.

Minutes later he returned with a pair of scissors and a roll of twine. The wall across from our bed is large and has two windows. Todd strung twine from one curtain rod to the other curtain rod, in between the windows. He made three swags with the twine and then hung all of the cards onto the swags. "Perfect. This is just perfect." I went a step further and taped up some of my favorite pictures from our recent vacation to San Diego.

I also began to flip through some of my magazines and started to cut out key words and phrases to adhere to the wall. I printed out 8.5 x 11 inch pieces of paper with positive affirmations:

"Thank you for my healing,"

"I am healed,"

"I feel wonderful,"

"I shall overcome."

These affirmations were then taped throughout our house, in the office, bathroom, kitchen and the bedroom.

I began to see this as one big vision board. I was determined to stay as positive as I could, especially now, since I would soon be starting chemo and had no idea what to expect.

Todd's Take

The mailbox was full everyday with cards, letters and well wishes from our friends and family. When Luci was sitting on the bed going through all the cards, I knew seeing them constantly would be a great motivator for her. She needed to be reminded of how much she had impacted everyone.

It also helped me realize we had a huge supportive network. Nieces' and nephews' artwork took up another wall. If nothing else, it certainly brightened up our master bedroom.

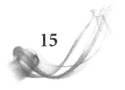

15

The Phone Call

For the very first time I felt as though I had been given a sign from above saying that it was going to be okay.

Wednesday, I prepared myself for my first chemotherapy appointment; it was for the following day. The only information I had been given was at my first post-surgical appointment: "Set aside six hours for the procedure." Knowing this, I packed a bag with reading material and my meditation CDs. For reading, Rita had thoughtfully brought a variety of inspirational books by Louise Hay to me when I was in the hospital. I added a few to my bag.

I was particularly attracted to a coloring book on mandalas. *Mandala* is a Sanskrit word that means "circle."

The Phone Call

In the Buddhist and Hindu religious traditions, their sacred art often takes a mandala form. In various spiritual traditions, mandalas may be employed for focusing attention of aspirants and adepts. It was used as a spiritual teaching tool for establishing a sacred space, and as an aid to meditation and trance induction. As a yoga instructor, these ideas and activities were important to me professionally, and now, even more important to me personally.

No longer were our lives a relatively simple schedule: to and from work daily during the week and planned or unplanned enjoyable weekend "adventures." Each week—almost 24/7—required a complex schedule involving Todd's business commitments and my recovery program. To this end, Todd worked to finalize our home schedule to coordinate visits with members of our families … Who would be coming to care for me; when would they arrive; and how long would they stay with us?

Added to the mix, he also needed to make sure I would always have someone here who could take me to my weekly lab visits. And during my chemo, I would need to go into my primary care physician every week to have my CBC monitored. Since I live 30 miles from my oncologist, my primary care physician was more than accommodating with this requirement. With those arrangements finally made, we were as ready as could be expected for this unknown phase of my journey.

Wednesday evening I received a phone call from the Visiting Nurses Association. The coordinator's name was

Connie. She informed me that my doctor, Dr. Hoeffer, had ordered a home nurse to be in charge of accessing and draining the fluid buildup in my right pleural sac. My nurse, whose name was also Connie, was scheduled to make her first house visit on Friday. Connie, the coordinator, then gathered the additional necessary information from me and we got the appointment scheduled.

Prior to hanging up, Connie said,

> Off the record, I too was diagnosed with Ovarian Cancer, Stage IV. I was given two months to live, and that was 20 years ago. When we received your case and I reviewed it, I knew it was God's will for me to share my story with you. Know there is hope and don't lose faith.

As I stood in my kitchen listening to Connie, tears filled my eyes and a numbing sensation cascaded through my entire body. I felt as if my legs were going to give out from under me. Filled with intense emotion, I managed to finally respond by saying simply, "Thank you."

She then said, "I wish you the best."

I hung up the phone then and just wept. It was another Moment—that sense of peace and calmness that overcame me—deep within my body. I was at ease—as I have mentioned, I don't believe in coincidence. For the very first time, I felt as though I had been given a sign from above saying that it was going to be okay.

Aunt Lu's Take

God knows how we all got through this so far. And we were given a miracle, and we didn't look back.

16

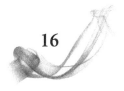

Round 1

Overall, I think all three of us felt a sense of relief. The first treatment was done and no significant side effects ... yet.

"Chemo day," Thursday, my alarm went off at 5:30 a.m. Although I was a little frightened about what was going to take place today, I refused to share these feelings with Todd or Aunt Lucy. I'm sure they were just as scared, but I needed to remain strong. While getting ready for this appointment and the ensuing treatment, I was determined to fix my hair and do my makeup. Personally for me, I knew how much better I felt in the hospital when I was dressed in my own clothes and had "done" my hair. Just brushing it and putting on a little eyeliner or lip shine did wonders for my morale. As I have made clear, I am a true believer in the importance of keeping a positive mindset, which in turn can affect a desired outcome. While I readied myself for the ordeal, Todd was busy making us lunch and getting the car packed.

At 6:45 a.m. we were loaded into the car and headed to my appointment. We arrived at 7:50 a.m. At 8:00 a.m., Dr. Schmitz's nurse, Karen, escorted us to the "Chemo" room. Karen was a petite woman with blonde, shoulder-length hair and a friendly, warm personality. When she smiled, her whole face lit up. She was so patient and empathetic. She asked me to choose any one of the ten teal recliners. I had a printout of the ingredients for the CR Support herbal supplements that our acupuncturist recommended I begin taking during my chemotherapy. I asked her if she could have Dr. Schmitz review it to see if I could take these herbs.

Karen took the document and said she would be glad to relay it to Dr. Schmitz and added that I would have an opportunity to discuss it later this morning during my routine examination. I then chose one of the recliners toward the end of the room, which allowed a little more room for Todd and Aunt Lucy to join me.

This would be my resting spot for the next six hours. Once settled, Aunt Lucy and Todd sat on either side of me. Karen rolled over a stand with three IV bags hanging from it and then returned with a portable roller cart and a stool. She took my vitals and then sat down in front of me and commenced to thoroughly cleanse and sterilize the area around my port. She asked if I was ready. I said, "Yes." She made the skin over the port taut and told me to take a deep breath. I automatically went into my yogic breathing.

The needle was successfully inserted into the port access. The pain was much more than that of a normal needle in the vein of your arm, but it quickly subsided. Karen then injected sodium chloride into the port to check the accessibility. She drew two vials of blood and started me on a bag of Benadryl and antibiotics while she ran a CBC. The other vial of blood would be sent off to the lab for a CA-125 blood marker reading.

(CBC stands for complete blood count. This test measures the number of red blood cells, white blood cells, the total amount of hemoglobin in the blood and your platelet count. All of these numbers are regularly monitored weekly during chemotherapy. Any dramatic changes to either of these numbers can affect whether or not your chemotherapy can continue or if a delay in treatment is necessary.

The CA-125, also known as cancer antigen-125, is a protein that is found at elevated levels in most ovarian cancer cells compared to normal cells. The CA-125 test assesses the concentration of CA-125 in the blood. The CA-125 marker will be checked at the start of every chemo treatment. This will help determine the activity of the cancer and the status of chemotherapy on the cancer.)

Round 1

Todd handed me my CD player with my yoga CD, *Crystal Healing Bowls*. The tones produced by crystal bowls are not just heard by the ear, you feel them in your body; certain tones affecting your energy centers (chakras) for healing, balancing and meditation. Within 15 minutes of the Benadryl IV, I was getting drowsy and shortly thereafter, I was out. I remember waking up and looking up at the clock; it said 11:30 a.m.! What happened to the time? I couldn't believe how the Benadryl affected me. Upon waking, Todd asked me how I was feeling.

Other than being really tired, I had, thus far, not experienced any side effects of the chemotherapy. I was about half way through the second bag.

I started feeling hungry. I sat up and was ready for one of those turkey wraps Todd had made for us. Neither Todd nor Aunt Lucy ate any lunch—it seemed they clearly were stressed out. Ironically, even though I was the patient and the one with cancer, it seemed as though I was less stressed than those caring for me. I knew I had to stay focused and remain in as much control as possible, which, I must admit, seemed to be harder and harder—less and less—each day … But my stubbornness and determination remained. I "soldiered" on.

During my IV session, Dr. Schmitz visited and spoke with me briefly noting that all seemed to be going well. She reviewed the herbal supplements and was fine with me taking them.

I finished my first round of chemotherapy at 1:30 p.m. Karen removed the bag, flushed my port with hep-lock and removed the needle. Again, not like a needle in your arm … you definitely feel it being pulled out with a firm grip. She then handed me a folder of information and briefly reviewed it with me.

Included were answers to many frequently asked questions about chemotherapy, its side effects and suggestions regarding diet due to some of the side effects. One of the forms Karen reviewed with me was the post-medication protocol that I was told to begin now. Two alternate regimens also were included which were to be implemented if nausea or intolerance to the first regimen occurred. My daily drug routine seemed to start at six in the morning and end at ten each evening.

Day One (Day of Chemo)
6:00pm   Compazine ½ to 1 tablet
10:00pm   Compazine ½ to 1 tablet

Day Two
6:00am   Compazine ½ to 1 tablet
8:00am   Dexamethasone 2 tablets with food
noon   Compazine ½ to 1 tablet
6:00pm   Compazine ½ to 1 tablet
10:00pm   Compazine ½ to 1 tablet

Day Three
6:00am	Compazine ½ to 1 tablet
8:00am	Dexamethasone 2 tablets with food
noon	Compazine ½ to 1 tablet
6:00pm	Compazine ½ to 1 tablet
10:00pm	Compazine ½ to 1 tablet

Day Four
6:00am	Compazine ½ to 1 tablet
8:00am	Dexamethasone 2 tablets with food
noon	Compazine ½ to 1 tablet
6:00pm	Compazine ½ to 1 tablet
10:00pm	Compazine ½ to 1 tablet

I must admit, I was frankly overwhelmed by all this information. Thankfully, we had the regimens, hard copy, and she recommended some vitamin supplements to help minimize and possibly prevent neuropathy. These supplements included B6, B12, B-Complex, Iron supplement, Calcium with Vitamin D and a multi-vitamin. Glutamine powder was also suggested to help minimize and possibly prevent joint and muscle pain, fatigue and neuropathy.

With the post-therapy interview done we gathered all of my "stuff" and left the office. On the way home, we stopped at Natural Grocers to buy the recommended vitamins. In addition to these supplements, I also added Mangosteen and Kombucha to my new, daily regimen.

"You are going to be fine Lucille, you hear me? ..."

Mangosteen is a tropical fruit that originates in East Asia. One of its biggest advantages is the presence of antioxidants to help strengthen the body's immune system. My immune system was in for the fight of its life, subjected as it would be for the next five months to a regimen of chemotherapy. Kombucha is an effervescent tea beverage, which can help detoxify and energize the body, clearly an important weapon also for the next five months' fight.

My main focus—and intense mind-set—as I began chemotherapy was to ensure I could maintain my strength during that next five months. I had already lost 14 pounds, which was over ten percent of my body weight before I was diagnosed with cancer. I did not have any weight to spare. I was afraid the chemotherapy was going to cause me to lose further, which could potentially jeopardize the long-term goal of the therapy. I was grateful that my appetite had returned to normal, so I needed to maintain my caloric intake and even possibly increase it to help regain the lost weight.

Thursday evening went rather well. I really didn't feel any different. Once again Todd was so right on when it came to keeping me on track with my medication. We decided to post the first medication protocol and check off every time that I took a pill. This really made a difference, making sure I was getting my medication at the proper times. In addition, I began my herbal supplements.

Overall, I think all three of us felt a sense of relief. The first treatment was done and no significant side effects … yet.

Friday morning was a sad day for me. Aunt Lucy was flying back to Utah this afternoon. I could tell she was nervous this morning knowing that she was leaving today. I remained strong, and did not want to show any fear, because I knew this would have made it that much harder for her. I reassured her I was okay and would be fine. Todd's Mom, Sue, was scheduled to arrive on Monday.

Aunt Lucy and I embraced, and she said, "You are going to be fine Lucille, you hear me? I will be back in three weeks. I love you." A few tears filled my eyes as I smiled back at her. Todd carried her luggage to the car and they were gone.

I received a call from Judy, another nurse who worked for Dr. Schmitz, with the results of my CA-125. My marker was at 4472. This meant nothing to me at this Moment, as I had no idea what was considered normal.

Judy continued. "Don't be concerned right now with the number, our goal is to get it within the normal range by the end of your sixth treatment." I asked what the normal range was and she told me under 20! I was dumbfounded. Could this really happen? I was mentally drained. Staying strong in the face of information like this was, to put it mildly, stressful beyond belief.

I spent much of Friday on the couch watching television and dozing in and out of sleep. I spent some time reading through all of the information Karen had given me.

Todd's Take

Luci's first treatment was uncomfortable for me. We were back in a sterile hospital environment, and I knew it had to be done. While Luci was hooked up to the chemo drip, I restlessly thumbed through old magazines and tried to get out to the cafeteria as much as possible. Fortunately, Aunt Lu was there and Luci was out cold, thanks to the Benadryl.

Thank God for the drug regimen printout. With everything else going on, the last thing I needed was to cause Luci any adverse reactions due to me forgetting her meds and another forty mile drive back to the ER. I paid complete attention when Karen walked us through the instructions.

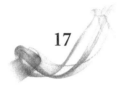

Cruella DeVille

I was starting to feel the effects of the chemo as my energy level began to drop, but I still couldn't let go of the idea of going to a Halloween party.

In our household Halloween is our favorite time. It was in October 2004 when Todd and I realized there was something more than being acquaintances with our mutual friends Chris and Aimee. Aimee and I had decided to host a Halloween party—a party that had been in the planning for many months. Our creative juices had been at work during the previous year—having fun was at the top of the list.

We had a great time planning and designing the details all that time. We would incorporate a murder mystery theme. Martha Stewart influenced our visual theme including making our own tomb stones for the front yard, skeleton lanterns, cobwebs made with yards and yards of cheese cloth and, of course, table settings and food. Time passed quickly and Halloween 2004, was upon us. I must say, Aimee's house looked like a page from Martha Stewart's *Living Magazine.* She would have been proud!

With the effort we put into it, this party was very important to me. I had such a great time planning and creating it with Aimee, yet when the day came, my husband at the time, would not even support my efforts by attending. This was yet another wedge that came between us. Despite this disappointment, our party was a success ... in more ways than one. The bonus for me was that it ended up not being tricks or treats ... Todd had formally entered my life. First as a friend, later as a husband.

Fast forwarding, this year was no exception. Todd and I were drawn to costumes for couples and themes involving cartoon characters. In the years past, we made a great Popeye and Olive Oil and Daphne and Shaggy. This was just a great way to have fun and bring out the kid from within. Pre-surgery, pre-ovarian cancer in our lives, we had already decided on our costumes, Cruella de Ville from *101 Dalmatians* and her henchman. I designed and made a Dalmatian print fur coat for the costume.

Now, with one of my favorite times of the year fast approaching, I was starting to feel the effects of the chemo as my energy level began to drop—I still couldn't let go of the idea of going to a Halloween party. Any Halloween

Cruella DeVille

party. I decided to call the one and only restaurant in Bailey to see if they were doing anything for Halloween.

> *I was ready to show my spots ...*

I couldn't believe it.... They were having a Halloween party the next evening sponsored by the local Lions Club—an all-you-can eat spaghetti dinner followed by a Halloween contest at 8 p.m. My excitement grew. I thought this just might be possible.

My biggest concern was staying up late to be present for the judging. Due to my growing chemo-induced fatigue over the past two weeks, I was usually in bed by 9 p.m. This was perfect; the judging was being done at 8 p.m. I could do this. When Todd got home, I was so excited to share what I had discovered. He seemed a little hesitant at first, but I begged him and told him this was just what I needed. "I need little goals that I can reach." This was so important to me mentally, to keep up the fight.

A bit skeptical, Todd agreed to go. I was so happy that I called Ray and Sherri to see if they wanted to go with us. I also called another friend of mine, Sandy and her husband, Paul, to see if they would like to come out and play with us as well. Sandy and I had met at the yoga studio in Conifer where I taught and she was one of my students. We knew each other for about three years but our friendship had only begun to blossom in June 2010. Once again, I saw the larger picture, for there are no coincidences in life.

I continued to stay on schedule with my medication, which seemed to be working fine. I was not experiencing any dramatic physical side-effects. I was, however, noticing my fatigue level was increasing. My appetite was still very good and I took advantage of this. I rested most of the day to prepare myself for this evening. Sandy and Paul were coming to pick us up at 7 p.m. and Ray and Sherri were going to meet us at the restaurant. I was glad I began to get ready at 5 p.m. because it took me that long to get the "job" done.

I did not have a lot of energy, but I was determined to go. Not going was NOT an option. I was putting on the finishing touches when I noticed the shoes I had bought for the costume didn't fit. They were too big! All the weight I had lost over the past three weeks not only affected my clothes but now my shoes. Who would have thought? On to plan B; thankfully I had another pair of shoes that would work. Nothing would hold back Cruella de Ville!

Arriving at the Rustic Station, we found the atmosphere in the restaurant was relaxed but festive. For Bailey, Colorado, this was the "happening" spot. Keep in mind, Bailey is a town of maybe 3000 people. Choices for entertainment were limited, but what was offered was just fine. For me, I was elated to be dressed up and getting out of the house. During dinner the judges mingled with the guests. To do a little preliminary judging, no doubt.

At 8:00 the judging began, and guess what … "First place goes to Cruella de Ville." You've got to be kidding!!!!!

OMG. I can't even put into words the feeling within. I was doing a happy dance in my body and my mind. You would have thought I had just won the lottery. The first prize was a handcrafted lamp carved out of an Aspen tree by a local artist. This just goes to show a fighting mind-set and determination can truly have a positive impact, no matter how insignificant the reward may seem.

For me the greater lesson was not about getting dressed up and winning. The lesson was that, as I began this uncharted journey, I had to remain strong. I was determined to get through this. I had to keep on fighting. I had to be me.

Todd's Take

With all the stress of the last two weeks, it was nice to see Luci maintaining some stability. Halloween was not going to pass without her wearing her Cruella costume. I had to relent. As weak as she was, she was not going to let it go. When she came downstairs in the costume, she had to sit down for me get a photo. I must say, in her emaciated state, she brought the cartoon character to life; pale, thin, sunken cheeks and a fake cigarette holder set the tone.

When Luci won the costume contest, I knew the night out had all been worth the effort. She glowed with a sense of accomplishment, down but not out!

18

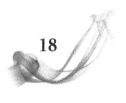

Sue

Sue is such an amazing woman. She is a spiritual healer and Reiki master

Three days since my first chemo treatment brought another physical change. I woke due to an ache in my knees and my lower legs. The sensation was similar to flu-like symptoms. My legs felt as though I had weights on them. I tried not to move around much but the pain was constant, dull and annoying. I did choose to take an Ultram, a pain pill I was given following my hysterectomy.

I spent most of the day in bed. I badly wanted to go sit in our hot tub. I thought the heat and jets on my legs would help reduce the aches. But since I had the drainage tube, the hot tub was off-limits. The next best alternative was to apply heat to my legs. I first tried applying a heating pad, which worked okay, but I later tried re-heatable heat wraps. This worked much better than the heating pad because they conformed better to my legs. I laid one of them just above my knees and then one just below my knees.

Between the pain medication and the heating wraps, the day was manageable. The nights that followed were a different story. The night sweats and the drainage tube made it very difficult to sleep. Many nights I would wake drenched and would have to change bedclothes. There were nights I was so uncomfortable that I would go downstairs and lay on the couch or try to sleep in my recliner.

Even though I was still very weak and not able to completely stand up straight, the pain and aches had subsided, and my mother-in-law, Sue, was flying in this morning. You hear stories of the dreaded mother-in-law … but I could not have been more blessed. From the first time she and I met, there was an instant connection. I knew that this Monday was going to be a good day.

We had so many things in common that we immediately developed a wonderful relationship. Sue is such an amazing woman. She is a spiritual healer and Reiki master. Her wisdom and intuitive insight is like no other. I couldn't wait for her to get here.

Sue spent a week with us. During this visit, she made meal after meal for us and packaged and froze many others for future use. In addition to cooking, she cleaned and caught up our laundry which had been neglected during

> *I know some may be leery of these techniques.*

the last three weeks. But the true gifts of her visit were more fundamental.

She had always known she had the special gift of clairvoyance. This however was profoundly expressed during her own fight with colon cancer 15 years ago.

Surgery removed 10 inches of her colon and was followed by chemotherapy and radiation.

Sue told me that being diagnosed with cancer was by far the toughest challenge she has ever dealt with in her life, but for her it was also one of her greatest gifts. Without this life experience, she would not have gained the knowledge and insight to help others. I so knew that her presence during this week would be not only healing for me, but insightful in sharing her expertise as someone close to me who has walked the cancer path.

Every morning she performed cleansings of my aura, spirit and soul on spiritual and astral levels. Sue also smudged our home and asked for assistance from her "team" and from my angels and guides to remove all negative and dark energies. She made it a point to share as much as she could from her cancer experience, so that I would have these tools available to me during the next several months. Sue continued this energy work and Reiki throughout my chemo treatment.

I know some may be leery of these techniques. I respect that. For Sue and me both, our bodies were dying. All I ask of you, my reader, is to be open to the many different healing modalities that exist and are used by many. When all that remains is Hope, embrace it. It is your life line.

Sue's Take

How I reacted to the call "Luci has cancer"… Shock. My mind went back 13 years ago to all that I had to experience. We never want our children to ever have to experience this. I went to my garden and I sobbed, not for me but for Luci and for Todd. I was angry. I could feel Todd's fear.

I am a Spiritual Counselor and I:
1. *Called on my guides, Crow, angels, masters, Christ and God.*
2. *I was in prayer every day, sending energy to both of them.*
3. *I smudged each day to remove old energy and fear. My intent was to create a space of positive energy where Luci could be healed in the love and light of all the guides and angels that were there to help*
4. *I know how powerful prayer is, and hands-on healing of Reiki and positive thoughts, and loving supportive people to be with you.*

*This was a very trying time for everyone.
Especially for the one that is ill and their mate.*

I thank God that I had the experience and knowledge to bring to Luci. I learned so much of healing in my experience of having colon cancer.

19

Burton

***I may have been down both physically and mentally,
but these outings reminded me of all the things
I needed to live for.***

Sue's week with us had been a Godsend. The following Monday was a tough day, because I had to say goodbye to her. Todd took her to the airport and I stayed home spending most of the day in bed. Within six hours of Sue's departure, my father-in-law, Burton, arrived. Todd's scheduling arrangements—arrangements guaranteeing that someone would be with me at all times—were working like a charm. I was really happy to see Burton, not only for myself, but for Todd. I knew he was really looking forward to seeing his dad. Todd, too, needed some TLC— Burton's arrival was just what my partner in life needed.

Burton was scheduled to spend the next week with us. During the evenings I would go to bed around 8 p.m.—I was just so tired. This gave Todd and his dad much needed time together. During the day, Todd would schedule calls with his business, and his dad would help out around the house and take me to my lab appointments.

Burton was scheduled to leave on the 14th of November and Aunt Lucy was to fly in that afternoon. Unfortunately, that was not to be. She had come down with a flu-like illness. I was paranoid about getting sick with chemo affecting my immune system, so I refused to allow anyone to come into our home with an illness. Aunt Lucy was rescheduled for a later time, and, thankfully, Burton was able to extend his visit with us for another week. This change of plans also gave us the opportunity to get to know one another a little better, and we found a common bond—the thrill of the shopping hunt. During my time home, now about a month, I spent a great deal of my day on the Internet. Before my diagnosis, I was no stranger to it. I would often get lost probing its depths. If there was a sale, forget it … I could spend three to four hours just surfing.

My greatest weakness is Kohl's department store. Not only is it easy to maneuver through their website, their marketing strategies are unsurpassed. They constantly send you 15, 20, 30 percent-off coupon codes and actually pay you to shop there in the form of "Kohl's Cash." Generally, I am not interested in applying for store credit cards. Kohl's is the exception. Okay, okay, I confess—I am a Kohl's junky.

Burton, on the other hand, had never been to Kohl's. This was my chance to recruit yet another loyal follower.

Thursday morning sitting at the kitchen table with my laptop, I, of course, was on the Kohl's website. This week happened to be a "Power Shopping Sale" week with up to an additional 30 percent off purchases. As luck would have it, I had in my possession, a 30 percent coupon. As I perused the web pages, Burton commented on how nice the flannel sheets have been to sleep on during his visit with us. Apparently that was not his experience at home. "Does Kohl's have flannel sheets?"

"Oh yes, and they're on sale right now." Burton didn't say much, but I know his interest had been piqued.

"This store practically paid us to shop."

I asked him if he wanted to get out of the house for a while. Personally, I could sure use a change of scenery. He agreed. He too thought a change of scenery would be good. We went to lunch and then headed to Kohl's.

Our shopping experience was a success for both of us. Burton found a set of flannel sheets, and I, of course, needed to add to my lounging attire. As the clerk rang up our purchases, the total bill was $58.79, a total savings of $62.00. In addition, since our purchases were over $50, we received a ten dollar Kohl's Cash voucher. Final cost for his flannel sheets was $17.78.

There was a puzzled look on Burton's face. As we left the store, he chuckled, "I have never witnessed such a thing. This store practically paid us to shop."

Three days later it was necessary once again to visit Kohl's; this time to take advantage of the Kohl's Cash. I convinced Burton that it was really necessary to have two sets of flannel sheets. This way he would always have a clean set on the bed while the other set is in the laundry. Final cost of this second pair of flannel sheets was $10.44! Burton had been initiated into the Kohl's devotee club!

It was great to get out of the house and do normal things. I may have been down both physically and mentally, but these outings reminded me of all the things I needed to live for. After many months of refusal, I am happy to report, the gold and maroon credit card is now in Todd's wallet … and I hope in Burton's.

Burton's Take

When Todd first informed me of Luci's cancer, I was very surprised. My first thought was, "How unfair for both of them." Todd had not been married and finally found the right one … and "Now This."

It was decided after Luci got out of the Hospital, she would need someone to stay with her during treatments. The family of both of them would come into play. I asked him to put me on the list and let me know the dates I would be needed.

My stay was going to be a week. Upon my arrival, I got the feeling everything was going to work out for the best. Where this came from, I have no idea. I did not know what the requirements would be but had decided I would do whatever it took. It turned out I was to be cook, partner but mostly chauffeur. The relatives prior to my arrival had cooked and stocked the freezer with food.

They had flannel sheets on the bed and I had never slept on these before. I made mention to Luci I was not going home without a set of them. Then the search began on her part. I have no idea how she could get so many discounts using her account and coupons. We headed to Denver for the shopping spree at Kohl's. We made the agreement she would take care of the purchase and I would reimburse her.

When all was said and done, I thought, "Kohl's is going to pay her to take them out of the store."

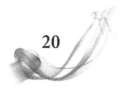

20

My Office Family

***As I greeted and hugged everyone, I jokingly said,
"You can't get rid of me that easy."***

On November 9th it had been one month since I had been in my office. It had been just a little over four weeks since my surgery—five months since I noticed the bump on my rib. I really needed to see my staff. With my new companion, I was ready to venture out. Burton and I headed into town. Our first stop was for lunch, with my office next. We arrived in the early afternoon.

When I left the office one month ago, what seemed to be just another ordinary departure turned into something totally unexpected. How are my co-workers going to react when they see me now? Did they ever think I would step foot in the office again? I had that classic nervous feeling of apprehension in my stomach as we entered the elevator and pressed "2."

The doors opened, we exited the elevator and entered the reception room. No one knew I was coming. As my eyes connected with Debbie at the front desk, my appearance startled her. She jumped slightly in her chair. Her eyes lit up and a huge smile appeared on her face. There was a similar expression with my other co-workers as I entered through the patient door and made my way around the front desk. Burton quietly took a seat in the reception area and waited for me.

Debbie and I have a special friendship and my unexpected illness hit her the hardest among the staff. She and I embraced each other and began crying. Others stood around, but knew not to approach us. We just held each other and cried.

I do believe seeing me with their own eyes, gave my staff hope of my return.

The fear and uncertainty felt by all, was unmistakable. For the past 17 years, I have been referred to as "the glue" that keeps this practice together. I wasn't about to let them down. As I greeted and hugged everyone, I jokingly said, "You can't get rid of me that easy."

I then made my way back to my office. Finding the glass door closed which was no surprise, I opened it and entered. Now alone, I sat in my chair and began to cry softly. Amazingly, sitting there in "my" space, isolated from the rest of the group, all my fears and worries seemed to disappear. I was temporarily removed from reality into a place of safety, comfort and peace. I closed my eyes and allowed these feelings to encompass my inner self. It was a quick return to my life, pre-diagnosis. I needed to know that my personal space and my co-workers were still there, waiting for me.

My visit was a success, both for me and my staff, and Burton and I left around 3 p.m. Although my visit today was emotionally draining, I do believe seeing me with their own eyes, gave my staff hope of my return. And, needless to say, it gave me that hope also … I wasn't planning on leaving.

Burton's Take

Luci had not been to her office in quite some time; she wanted to go in for a visit. We headed down the hill to Denver to complete this task. When we arrived, it was like old home week. I just got a magazine and sat in the waiting room.

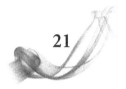

The First Noticeable Changes of Chemo

For the first time, the realization really set in;
I was going to lose my hair.

As each day passed with my regular, continuing chemo treatment, I could feel a subtle increase in fatigue, but, on the positive side, as time went on I was able to get around much better since the surgery.

On the fourteenth day of chemo, as usual I was sitting in my recliner watching TV and Todd and Burton were at the kitchen table. I ran my fingers through my hair and there "it" was. What a shock. The Moment had arrived that I had been dreading since my diagnosis. My hair was beginning to fall out. In between my fingers were strands of my hair. For the first time the realization really set in; I was going to lose my hair. In fact, it had begun!

When I heard the word chemotherapy, I automatically thought, "Am I going to lose my hair?" Even though I was told it was inevitable, there was something inside of me holding onto the tiniest glimmer of hope that maybe, just maybe, my body would respond differently; my hair would be spared. This was not to be; the stark reality was, I was going to lose my hair! I was going to be bald! There was the damning evidence in my fingers.

"What's Wrong?"
- Rita

Devastated, I got up from my recliner and went upstairs. I needed to be alone. I went into my bedroom, closed the door, got into bed and began to cry. I needed to talk to Rita right away. I picked up the phone and called her. In her usual cheerful, upbeat voice she greeted me. "Good morning, Luci, how are you feeling?"

I replied, "Ok." Rita knew me better than anyone else. She could see right through my response. Tone reveals all.

"What's wrong?" she immediately replied. Tears filled my eyes and I was unable to speak for a moment, but then managed in my tragic tone, "My hair is falling out."

"Luci, listen to me, we talked about this and we knew this was going to happen. This is only temporary. You need to stay focused and know that the chemo is obviously working. Yes, it's killing your healthy cells that allow your hair to grow, but it is also killing those cancer cells."

The First Noticeable Changes of Chemo

Rita always had a way with words. Whenever I was feeling down or upset about something, all I had to do was call her. She was able to change my mindset completely and put me into a better mood.

Losing my hair from chemo is truly a weird experience. When I pull on it there is no sensation; it just comes out. It reminds me of when I was a little girl and I got into fights with my brothers. Having my hair pulled was a regular event. If you've ever had your hair pulled really hard, it almost makes a tearing sound, similar to ripping of a seam or tearing a piece of cloth. Strangely, I could hear it within my head; but the hair actually would never come out. Now, as I sat there on my bed and ran my fingers through my hair, there was no such sensation. The hair just came out and there was no pain at all.

I was now hesitant to brush it or wash it frequently. I was hoping to hold onto it for as long as I could, but over time, more and more strands were coming out, especially during the night when I was sleeping. There was increasing baldness on the top of my head and in the temple area. I'm sure it was the friction on the pillow due to sleeping on my side; the effect was similar to that of a baby.

A bandanna now became the primary styling tool for my hair. Quite simple and basic, I just put one on, leaving what little bit of hair I had left sticking out of the back of the bandanna, on the nape of my neck. This was no different from coordinating my loungewear. It fit right into my routine; I just had an additional accessory to coordinate.

I remained committed to showering every day and getting dressed despite my ever-increasing fatigue. Not only did it make me feel better, it helped me hold onto what little bit of "normalcy" Todd and I had left. I may be going bald, but I would do it in style.

Aunt Lu's Take

At times I felt like I was going to have a meltdown. I would start to shake and cry. I had to take my Ativan religiously to control it.

Luci would send us pictures along the way as she was losing her hair.

I know she was trying to prepare us.

No matter what you feel or how much you love someone, it is so difficult to see and digest.

Somehow, you realize that a person's appearance doesn't matter, it is who they are that makes them so very very special.

22

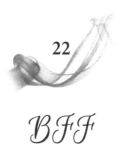

BFF

... she has been—and still is—my rock along with Todd, as we look into a very uncertain future.

Every woman needs a before, during and after friend. (Now, now, guy-readers, if you need one too, be my guest.) Rita is mine. We have been friends for over 20 years. We were both flight attendants (please, *not* stewardesses!) for Continental Airlines. We met through a mutual friend, another flight attendant, while on a three-day trip. We had the opportunity to fly together on the same crew, and then we were scheduled together again for another trip. We really seemed to hit it off, and, both of us being based in Denver, we thought it would be nice to get together during some off time with our husbands and go to dinner.

From the start, we had a lot of fun together and really enjoyed each other's company. In the airline industry there is a term referred to as "buddy-bidding." This term meant two flight attendants can bid the same schedule for a given month and would fly together on these trips. Rita and I decided we would do that for a month.

The nicest thing about buddy-bidding was that it removed the sense of awkwardness of not knowing who your crew was going to be for the next given time frame. Now you always knew at least one person on the crew. This also made layovers less lonely. Rita and I always had a blast. In fact, we continued to buddy-bid for the next two years.

We became inseparable. We were often referred to Lucy and Ethel, Frick and Frack, Betty and Wilma. We had a great time and loved our jobs. We flew in the late 80s and early 90s, well before 9/11. The airline industry was totally different; it was a great job to have then. We had great layovers with great people and (as I said) we did have a lot of fun; at times too much fun and maybe a little too much partying. At this time in our lives, I would not have traded it for anything. Rita and I became "grounded" so to speak, ending our flying careers in 1994 when Continental closed its hub in Denver.

Our professional careers together did not end there, however. Shortly after leaving Continental Airlines, we found ourselves working together once again, this time in a periodontal practice of all things. This was a huge change for both of us, having been glorified waitresses for the past eight years. The change was a bit scary for us, but we were ready for the challenge. To make a long story short, Rita and I continued to work together the next 18 years for Professional Periodontics and Implant Dentistry in Denver.

Needless to say, a very special friendship has developed over 20 plus years. Rita is the sister that I never had. And, as it can be with sisters, our friendship has lasted and grown through the many trials in each of our lives. We've helped each other through breakups, illnesses of our parents, the death of my father, divorces, marriages, loss of our beloved pets, and now, a life-threatening illness for one of us.

There is an intuitive sense that evolves between girlfriends. You know when the other one is in need of help, encouragement or just some space. This fight of mine will be no different than any of the other challenges she and I had been through. Since the first night in the ER, Rita has called every day to check in with me. On those few occasions where she had been out of town traveling on speaking engagements, and the time zones were not conducive to calling, she would check in via text messages.

As I have already made quite clear, she has been—and still is—my rock, along with Todd, looking into a very uncertain future. Thanks, Rita. You know how I feel. BFF.

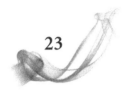

23

Round 2

At 1:30 p.m. I was done. Two down, four to go.

At 6:45 a.m. on November 18, Todd, Burton and I headed out to Dr. Schmitz's office for my second treatment of chemotherapy. We arrived at eight, were again greeted by Karen and the routine for pre-op was repeated. She cleansed the port site prior to access. Then, once the Huber needle pierced the port, Karen drew two vials of blood. One was needed to run my CBC, and the other was sent off for a CA-125 marker reading. Karen returned with the CBC and all was within the limits to proceed. She began with a Benadryl drip.

The side effects this time were not as dramatic as the first treatment. I was able to stay awake. Todd and Burton stayed with me until the Benadryl was completed to make sure that all was well.

Mentally, I needed my time with my girlfriends. Many, I know, think it would be great not to have to work and just stay home. Well, I'm here to tell you, it's not that great. All I wanted to do was to be at work. As with most things, I don't think we truly appreciate how much enjoyment and fulfillment we get from interaction with our co-workers, until we are away from them for an extended period of time. It was now a month plus.

All I wanted was to be at work!

For that reason, oddly enough, I looked forward to this chemotherapy session so that I could see my office "buddy," Debbie, and get a sense of reconnection to the practice again. She planned to visit me in the "Chemo Room" and be with me for the entire treatment. Her presence gave Todd and Burton the opportunity to spend some time together as well as go out and about, running errands.

It had been three weeks since I started chemo, and I was starting to experience dry, flaky skin. Three things, as a result, were on my shopping list: baby oil, Katy Perry's newest CD, *Teenage Dream*, and more bandannas, in a variety of colors.

Debbie's visit was truly a needed distraction from my well established routine. As I lay there subjected to the IV, and visiting with her, we were in our own little world, unaffected by anything around us and totally consumed with each other's presence.

At 1:30 p.m. I was done. Two down, four to go.

The drainage tube for my right lung was still required to assist in the elimination of fluid from my right lung. 400 ml (about a pint!) were being extracted twice a week.

But, after one treatment of chemotherapy, the bump on my rib was GONE!!!!!! Something's working.

The results of my CA-125 were in—it was cut by 75 percent. It was 1198. Huge !!!!!!!!!!!

Burton's Take

When it was time for her Chemo Treatment, I was a little apprehensive. Todd had to meet someone for lunch concerning business, so the three of us headed down the hill. I had never been a part of, or exposed to, anything like this.

As it turned out, I was the only one that had any concern. Todd and Luci took it as just part of the situation. Luci had a book and her CD player and was ready to be connected. There were a couple of other women there for the treatment. I stayed there for a while and listened to them talk. I again got that positive feeling. I hope it worked out for the other women as well as it did for Luci.

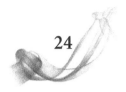

24

Are You Going to Eat That??????

*"My God, you ate more than we did.
I just can't believe it."*

I have had two chemo treatments and oddly enough my appetite was increasing. I don't know why or what was causing this, but I had to assume it was the chemo. This was a welcomed change, a definite positive in a generally negative outlook. As I had mentioned, I was determined to make sure I continued to eat normally to fuel my body and to give it as much energy as I could to kill the cancer.

During this time, a night visitor entered my life. My routine still included retiring early—with sleep occurring as soon as my head hits the pillow. Every evening close to midnight or in the very early morning, I was awakened by hunger pangs. I would have to make my way downstairs and eat another full meal. This usually occurred nightly around 1 am.

As each day passed, I continued to heal from the surgery and was becoming more restless. I yearned to get out of the house. One of the benefits of living in a small mountain town is the absence of crowds. This was more important than ever, because I continued to be hesitant to expose myself to large groups of people for fear of catching "something" and getting sick. Going out here in Bailey, avoided that danger pretty much.

One evening, Todd, Burton and I ventured out to one of the two restaurants we have here in Bailey. Chinese was our choice tonight. We ordered crab wontons as an appetizer, and each ordered an entrée. Soup preceded the entrée for each of us. By the time our entrees were delivered, both Todd and Burton's appetite had slowed down a bit. Not mine. I continued to eat until my plate was empty. I looked over at Todd's plate; there lay an uneaten spring roll. "Are you going to eat your spring roll? Cause if not, can I have it?" Todd just smiled and handed it over. After I consumed the coveted spring roll, I placed my fork down on my plate and slid it over to the right—I was finished. My father-in-law looked over at my empty plate and then turned to me and then Todd with a look of amazement.

Burton has a bit of a mid-western, southern drawl and a very dry sense of humor. He looked over at me again and said, "I dang near thought you were going to eat the plate. My God you ate more than we did. I just can't believe it." To this day, he still tells this story.

Burton's Take

When we got our dinner, it was not on a plate, it was on a platter. The food sure looked and tasted very good but a lot of it. I could not clean up my plate. Luci kept eating until her plate was clean.

While she was eating, I kept wondering, "Where is she putting all this food. I just knew she had a hollow leg."

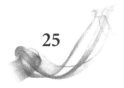

Anger—Part of the Grieving Process

***I wanted to throw every single glass object against
the wall just to hear the crashing sound
of something breaking.***

Up to this point in time, for the most part, I felt like I was handling this life-changing event fairly well. Until today …

What started out to be what I have now come to accept as a normal day became anything but normal. Today was Tuesday, November 23rd, the fifth day following my second chemo. I'm now five weeks post surgery.

As I awoke, I found that I was on my stomach and lying across the bed on Todd's side. I rolled over and untangled myself from my oxygen tubing. I sat up then and started to get out of bed. The achiness was already starting in my legs and knee joints, identical to what I experienced after my first chemo treatment. But as I sat up I could feel tightness in my upper back and right shoulder. This was obviously due to the drainage tube in my rib. I just felt "a bit off."

I finished the process of getting out of bed, pulled on a robe and went downstairs. There on the counter, wrapped in plastic wrap was a toasted bagel sandwich. This had become one of my favorite breakfast treats. An egg over hard, topped with a slice of ham, and cheese melted on top, all neatly sandwiched between a whole-wheat bagel, thin.

What a wonderful surprise Todd left me prior to leaving for work. It did not affect my mood, however. My focus remained on the tightness which had evolved into a horrible pain in my upper back and shoulder, and there was the developing achiness in my leg; I couldn't even enjoy his edible token of affection. I was in pain, in a horrendous mood and feeling very pissy.

I just felt a bit off ...

I sat in my recliner and ate my sandwich. After I had finished, I put my plate on the coffee table and reached for our wedding photo album, which was sitting next to my plate, and I began to look through it as my dark mood deepened. I became very upset and began to cry because, as I flipped through the pictures, what set me off were the pictures of my niece, Brooklyn. This beautiful, precious child ... I have to see her grow up!

To be quite frank, this day was already FUCKED up. I had such a feeling of anger and rage within me. I looked down at my plate on the coffee table and then all around our living room and dining room. I wanted to throw every single glass object against the wall just to hear the crashing sound of something breaking. For some quite irrational reason, at this very Moment, that sound, I thought, would help bring me comfort. I pondered this angry, impulsive thought for a Moment and was prepared to act it out, when sanity struck. Someone would have to clean the stupid mess up! There was no one else but me.

If I didn't have to clean up the aftermath, I would have followed through …

Okay, so we've all either heard or read about it … Being diagnosed with cancer is a traumatic, life-changing event and it's normal and natural to grieve. By going through the grieving process, we are given time to reflect and find new strength that will enable us to continue life's journey and regain peace-of-mind.

It wasn't until after this emotional episode, that I realized I was in fact, grieving.

As evening approached—and with it, reason, along with less pain—my emotional state had improved greatly.

26

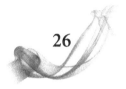

A Sense of Normalcy

***Six weeks post surgery, I was on my own
and able to drive once again.***

The house was still. For the first time since my diagnosis, we were alone. Todd's dad, Burton, had returned home three days after my 2nd chemo treatment and it was a relief for family not to be here. It was a paradox. Our families volunteered to help us in our hour of need, and we needed their help badly during those trying weeks. We welcomed them and were immensely grateful. Yet there was a sense of relief in their absence that both Todd and I felt. Yes, it had been great to have family here to help us but with that also came a feeling of obligation. They are family, but they were still guests in our home.

Things do have a way of working out for the highest good. Aunt Lucy's flu may have prohibited her from

What a freeing experience!

coming to care for me, a clear negative, but it also provided much needed alone time for Todd and me. Our home isn't large in the first place, but it seemed to have become smaller with every well-intentioned visit.

Today was another milestone. Six weeks post surgery, I was on my own and able to drive once again. Woo-Hoo! This was the first time since my diagnosis, and I drove myself to my primary care physician for my routine blood draw. What a freeing experience! I could finally depend on myself to get around. Today was an awesome day.

While Todd was at work, I also took advantage of this time alone to check on resources that were available to cancer patients. I was particularly interested in a flyer I saw at Dr. Schmitz's office about "Nicki's Circle." It was a local support group in the Denver area sponsored by the Colorado Ovarian Cancer Alliance.

On their website I learned how to register, the frequency of their meetings and their locations. I wanted to expand my understanding and knowledge about this disease and learn what others have experienced as well as treatment options.

What a wonderful way for Todd and me to educate ourselves and to share our feelings with others dealing with similar issues. It just so happened their next meeting in central Denver was scheduled for December 9th, less than two weeks from now.

My Mom was scheduled to spend the first two weeks of December with me. This would also be a great opportunity for her. During my continued Internet searches, among a wealth of material, I came across a program called *Look Good, Feel Better* which was sponsored by the American Cancer Society. This program is a workshop which teaches beauty techniques to female cancer patients to help them combat the appearance-related side effects of chemotherapy. There were several locations throughout metro Denver. As I continued my search, they too were offering a workshop during her visit. Putting both dates on my calendar, I knew that Mom would want to attend and learn everything she could.

This time alone also gave Todd and me a chance to spend time with Rita and Michael, as couples and as friends. In years past, Rita and Michael would spend Thanksgiving with us. This year, the tables were turned. Todd and I went to their home. Rita had everything ready. Todd stepped in as her prep chef, chopping and sautéing the onions, celery and garlic for the dressing. The synchronicity between the two of them was amazing. The aromas were fabulous—I loved it that my appetite was looking forward to this feast.

Michael and I just sat at the bar, drank wine and watched. Our visit together brought back memories of how things used to be, and how I longed for this to be once again. In due time….

Only one minor casualty … the garlic press.

Mom's Take

After some chemo, she started to lose her hair.
Little by little she got thin and frail.
A specimen of perfect health no longer.

I was so sad to see her lying in bed and then the shock to see her bald, something I will never forget. I cried by myself when I was alone and prayed and prayed the chemo would killing that fucking disease.

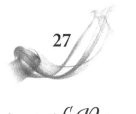

27

Power of Prayer

"I was told you needed to have these.
They should be placed near your bed."

There are several documented studies on the healing of disease and illness through prayer. From the very beginning of this journey, prayer became an integral part of my daily life. My name was added to several prayer chains throughout the community. I also wrote a letter to my fellow yogis asking for their prayers and intentions during their yoga practices.

I received a package from Sue today. I had no idea how much of an impact this package would have on me. When I opened it, there was a beautiful cherry wood box with a golden clasp. I lifted it and opened the box. The inside was lined with red velvet and nestled within the velvet lining were two sachets, one filled with frankincense and the other with myrrh. In the center was a glass bottle filled with liquid and shaved pieces of gold.

At first, I wasn't sure what the gifts represented. I called Sue to thank her. Sue said,

---

"... I need your help ..."

She went on to explain the significance of each of the contents. Myrrh is supportive of the immune system. It helps in the fighting of infection and helps to get rid of negative energy. The frankincense helps to build the immune system and helps to overcome depression; the gold represents the fact that I am surrounded and protected by a golden shield, which will allow me to receive a healing from Spirit.

There was also a ceramic statue of the Blessed Mother with child. In the bottom of the package was a white envelope. The envelope contained two prayer cards, *The Miracle Prayer* and *Prayer to Saint Peregrine*, the cancer saint.

At the bottom of *The Miracle Prayer* in small-italicized text it said, *Say this prayer faithfully, no matter how you feel. When you come to the point where you sincerely mean each word, with all your heart, something good spiritually will happen to you. You will experience Jesus, and HE will change your whole life in a very special way. You will see.*

The Miracle Prayer

Lord Jesus, I come before you just as I am. I am sorry for my sins, I repent of my sins, please forgive me.

In your name I forgive all others for what they have done against me. I renounce Satan, the evil spirits and all their works. I give you my entire self, Lord Jesus, now and forever. I invite you into my life, Jesus. I accept you as my Lord, God and Savior. Heal me, change me. Strengthen me in body, soul and spirit.

Come, Lord Jesus, cover me with your precious blood, and fill me with your **Holy Spirit. I love You, Lord Jesus. I Praise You, Lord Jesus. I thank you, Jesus**. I shall follow you every day of my life. Mary, my mother, Queen of Peace, St. Peregrine, the cancer saint, and all you Angels and Saints, please help me.

Amen

A Prayer to St Peregrine for One Suffering from Cancer

Dear St. Peregrine,
I need your help.
I feel so uncertain of my life right now.
This serious illness makes me long for
a sign of God's love.
Help me to imitate your enduring faith
when you faced the
Ugliness of cancer and surgery.
Allow me to trust the Lord
the way you did in this Moment
of distress. I want to be cured,
but right now I ask God for
the strength to bear the cross in my life.
I seek the power to proclaim
God's presence in my life
despite the hardship, anguish,
and fear I now experience.
O Glorious St. Peregrine,
be an inspiration to me
and petitioner of these needed graces
from our loving Father.
Amen

From this Moment forward, I prayed these two prayers along with the Rosary every day.

Sue's Take

After the initial shock and rage, I pulled myself together and started to pray. I am a Reiki Healer, I called on my masters to set in motion, what we could do. First I wanted to clear the fear from Todd and Luci—sacred space if you will. We needed God, our angels and positive loving energy.

I talked to Todd each day on Luci's progress. One day he said "Mom—Luci called from the hospital at 7a.m., after her surgery and asked where the #^%& are you?" We each laughed, which released the stress and I told him Luci will be fine, she is a fighter and she needs to be. Remember, the mind is feeling fear, pain, and why me, I did all the right things. Why??

I live in Kansas, they in Colorado. I went to help in any way that I could, cook, clean and help each of them.

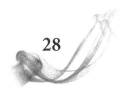

Mother and Daughter Time

I don't care how old you are ... There are times in our lives when we just need our Mom.

My Mom and my older brother Frank were flying in today. I was so happy they were coming and was eager to see them. Frank was spending just an extended weekend with us, but Mom was staying for 15 days! My Mom and I talked every day by phone, but this was the first time seeing her since my surgery. It seemed ages ago. So many things had changed over the past eight weeks. Todd went to the airport to pick them up while I stayed at home.

At 1:30 p.m. Tara and Rafferty jumped off our bed and ran down the stairs. They knew before I did that they were here. Then I heard the sound of the car drive up. They're here!! I was filled with mixed emotions. I was so excited to see both of them, at the same time I was scared to have them see me skinny, pale and bald.

The front door opened. "Luci?"

"I'm up here, Babe."

I could hear the creaking of the hardwood stairs. "Lucille?"

"I'm in here, Ma." My Mom slowly opened the bedroom door. I sat up in bed. As I looked to the door and saw my mother's face, I removed my bandana and began to cry. "I'm so ugly."

She came over to my bedside, wrapped her arms around me with her hands on my head and held me. "Shhhhhh, it's okay. We knew this was going to happen. It's only temporary, Lucille." She gently swayed back and forth with me in her arms, refusing to let go.

I don't care how old you are … There are times in our lives when we just need our Mom. No one else's words, touch or love will do.

My brother Frank does not do well with things like this. If he had his "druthers," he'd much rather change the subject or ignore it all together. I knew this was extremely difficult for him, but I was so happy to see him. He soon got over his aversion of the situation and we spent much of our time reminiscing about our childhood and the crazy things we used to do. We also did a lot of eating. Mom kept busy cooking all of our favorite Italian meals.

After arriving, Todd and Mom headed to the store, giving Frank and me some time to ourselves. His time would be short and we needed to make the best of it. During our conversation, I began to cry over losing my hair. Frank came over and hugged me. "You know I would do whatever I could for you, but this is something you need to do—only you can deal with. I would do it in a second, but I can't. You're alive. Your hair loss is only temporary."

Although our visit was short, our bond as brother and sister grew stronger and deeper.

For not really having anything to do—we had a pretty full calendar.

Mom stayed home with me while Todd drove Frank back to the airport. This gave us some time together to plan Mom's remaining time with me. For not having anything to do, we had a pretty full calendar over the next 11 days. Tomorrow would begin with a visit from Connie, dealing with my weekly fluid buildup followed by a stop at my primary care physician for a blood draw. Then we were introduced to Nicki's Circle and a meeting with ovarian cancer patients.

Todd met Mom and me at St. John's Cathedral, where Nicki's Circle holds their meetings. I was nervous at first, but that quickly diminished. Being surrounded by other ovarian cancer patients and survivors, helped to remove some of my fears. This support group was just that: extremely supportive, as well as being very informative.

At the conclusion of the meeting , we visited a table at the back of the room where there were brochures and informational pamphlets. Looking through that array of literature, I was pleasantly surprised to stumble upon an organization called "Life Spark Cancer Resources."

This organization's focus is matching Reiki and Healing Touch practitioners with individuals with cancer. As a Reiki master myself, this was a wonderful discovery. I had no idea such an organization existed. I couldn't wait to get in touch with them. This enforced my belief in the necessity of incorporating holistic therapies with western therapies, an idea not accepted by a significant fraction of practitioners of mainstream western medicine.

Attending this support group and the information I received was just the tip of the iceberg of things to come …

The following day, Mom and I attended the "Look Good … Feel Better" workshop. There were a total of six women participants in the workshop. It was led by two volunteer cosmetologists. Each cancer patient was given a handbook, illustrating how to apply makeup, with suggestions on which type of skin care products were best for your skin during chemotherapy treatment. In addition, we each received a large makeup bag filled with full-sized beauty products. These products were from Lancome, Estee Lauder, Clinique, Aveda and Origins, to name a few.

For me personally, I felt better after the workshop which I found to be informative and educational. Very useful, in other words, for someone who felt she needed all the help she could get with regard to her appearance.

The alarm went off at 6:00 a.m. Here we go again. Round three. Todd drove the three of us to my chemotherapy appointment. I was especially excited this morning. Today would also be my first session with Bob, a Reiki master and practitioner from Life Sparks Cancer Resource Center, the outfit I discovered in the literature at the ovarian cancer workshop.

Shortly after 10:00 a.m., Todd and my Mom went off to run some errands. I was content to be listening to my CDs and relaxing. This time alone also gave me an opportunity to color in my Mandalas coloring book. I know this may sound odd, being accused of a serious reverting to childhood would be hard to avoid, but I had so much fun coloring. What a therapeutic experience! It was as though all my worries and concerns were lifted from me during that time.

Todd and my Mom arrived back at 1:30 p.m. Treatment went according to plan; with one exception. My white blood count was dropping, heading to a critical level. I was sent home with a Neulasta injection, which I would need to have administered 24 hours after chemotherapy. Neulasta boosts your white blood cells and is commonly prescribed during chemo treatments. Without this injection, I would most definitely be at great risk.

We were now on our way to my Reiki appointment. As a Reiki practitioner, I knew of its the benefits. Being as ill as I was, created barriers for me—it prohibited me from fully engaging in performing Reiki on myself.

Reiki is a Japanese technique for stress reduction and relaxation that also promotes healing. Reiki treats the whole person, including body, emotions, mind and spirit. It creates many beneficial effects including relaxation and feelings of peace, security and well-being. Reiki has been effective in helping a wide variety of illnesses and maladies, and it works well in conjunction with medical treatments to relieve side effects and promote recovery.

What makes Reiki unique is that it works from a subtle level of our existence, where imbalance begins. As balance is regained, superficial symptoms often disappear, enabling the body's innate healing potential to be enhanced. Reiki can be a valuable addition to any treatment plan or well-being program. It doesn't matter if you are in the beginning stages or well-advanced, maintaining balance is critical to mental and physical health.

> *My body was overcome with a feeling of complete relaxation.*

We arrived just before 2 p.m. and Todd and Mom stayed in the car while I went into my session. When I entered, I was met with a friendly greeting by "Bob," a gray haired gentleman of medium build who looked to be in his mid to late 50s. I lay down on the massage table, face up and closed my eyes.

During my session, I remember seeing the colors lavender, pink and yellow in my mind's eye, and my body was overcome with a feeling of complete relaxation. The session was clearly beneficial, and I set up future weekly sessions with Bob.

On our way home, I felt really good about "things." I was half way through my chemo and the amount of fluid being extracted from my lung had begun to decrease; I was down to 250ml twice a week—approximately a pint of fluid a week. Progress was being made. It made me smile within. Now if only I could get rid of this tube by Christmas.

The remaining week or so with my Mom, before she had to return, was spent at home. She attended to my common, post-chemo ailments which hit like clockwork, three and five days after. During her last couple of days with us, she tidied up our house, changed our bedding, did laundry, and cooked non-stop, preparing meals for us to have until her next scheduled visit in February.

CA-125 had decreased 80% !!!!!!!! … 233. Wow!

29

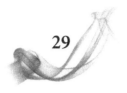

And You Are????????

**As I looked at his big brown eyes, I could tell;
he didn't know who I was.**

If you are or were a pet owner, you know how intuitive and smart pets are. Tara and Rafferty were no exception. They knew something was not right from the Moment I came home from the hospital and stepped through the door.

On any ordinary return home, both Tara and Rafferty would be whining and wagging their tails at the front door. They couldn't wait for the door to open and bombard us; each one of them trying to out-compete the other for our attention, love and affection. But today, Sunday, October 17th, when I first returned home from the hospital, was not an ordinary return. As I mentioned earlier, I was struggling not to shit myself and make it to the bathroom.

As Todd opened the door, and I made my way to the bathroom, both Tara and Rafferty just stood on either side of the door. It was as if they knew to keep the path free and clear for me. There was a different energy about them. This change in their behavior continued throughout my illness and initial recovery time. Rafferty, who is more "my dog" than Todd's, became very clingy. He was by my side all the time.

"Rafferty ... its Mama,"

Rafferty would take naps with me, lay under the computer desk when I was working, and he started sleeping on the floor next to my side of the bed. Even when I would shower in the morning, he had to be with me in the bathroom or he would start whining and scratching at the door. Rafferty was like the shadow that Wendy had sewn to the bottom of Peter Pan's feet!

I can't stress enough how important and therapeutic this was for me. On the flip side, I wasn't prepared for the heart wrenching experience that surfaced as my chemo treatments progressed.

Todd cautiously mentioned that I was beginning to resemble a Scooby-Doo cartoon villain with the patchy, thin hair. Although I knew this was extremely difficult for Todd to say, I was so thankful we hadn't lost our ability to communicate—and with humor sprinkled in.

I finally decided it was time to shave my head of what little strands of hair remained. We went to the bathroom and he lathered my head up with shaving cream. Gently, he proceeded to shave my head, removing the last stubborn strands of my once long, beautiful mane. We cried together as he rinsed the remaining shaving cream from my now barren scalp.

It will grow back … eventually. And at least I didn't resemble the Scooby Doo villain any longer.

When this daunting task was done, I must admit, I felt a sigh of relief. It was done; I was now officially bald. Thankful that I didn't smell like Old Spice, I left the bathroom and proceeded down our spiral staircase. Rafferty was lying next to my recliner. As I approached the bottom of the stairs, he sat up but didn't move. His little white head tilted to the right and he had a puzzled and confused look on his face. As I looked at his big brown eyes, I could tell; he didn't know who I was.

"Raffers, its MaMa." Once he heard my voice, he immediately came to the bottom of the staircase to greet me, wagging his tail enthusiastically. I knelt down, hugged him as tight as I could and sobbed.

Rafferty' Jake

It's been unsettling around here. So many people in and out. They are very nice to Tara and me—lots of scratches, walks and food ... but MaMa has something wrong. We don't know what it is, but have to watch out for her; to stay close to her. I know she needs me.

When she came down the stairs, I thought another stranger was in the house. The shiny head scared me a little. Then I heard the voice—my MaMa was the shiny head!

30

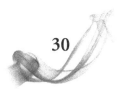

100.6

"There is definitely an infection here."

From all the literature I was given, the potential side effects of chemotherapy freaked me out and more than a bit. I had now completed three of my six chemotherapy treatments and have had minimal side effects. I couldn't help but contribute some of this to the herbal supplements I'd been taking since the start of the treatments. Things were going as well as could be expected ... until I got out of the shower.

As I was drying myself off, I noticed a little redness next to the drainage tube to the right of my belly button. Before showering, I covered the tubing and incision site, with a clear plastic adhesive patch just as Connie had taught me. With an increased risk of infection during chemotherapy, Dr. Schmitz's office recommended taking my temperature regularly. This was something I did every morning since chemotherapy had started. My temperature was 97.6. All is okay …

Later that evening I began to feel an achy sensation around the drainage tube. Removing the dressing the redness was still there, but the red area had become larger. Reaching for the thermometer, I once again took my temperature. Now it read 100.6. Oh My God! This is bad. I had been instructed to contact Dr. Schmitz if my temperature reached 100.5 or above.

I immediately called to Todd. He dialed her office, which went directly to the answering service. He was placed on hold while the operator paged the doctor. Nancy, one of Dr. Schmitz's' nurses, responded. Todd then handed me the phone and I explained my symptoms. As soon as I finished, she told me I should go to the ER right away.

Having gone to the hospital multiple times prior and knowing the outcome, I decided to go upstairs and pack a bag. While I did that, Todd put the dogs in their kennel in the garage and we were on our way.

Once again, on a Sunday evening, we wound down the hill and headed to the ER arriving around 9:30 p.m. I had lost count of how many trips we had made to this hospital over the last three months. But I can tell you, when the staff recognizes you and you're on a first name basis with them, it's been TOO, TOO many.

My temperature was taken upon admission. It was rising; 101.6. I was brought back to a room. Dr. Brent was the ER physician on duty. He examined the drainage tube. "There is definitely an infection here." As he gently pushed around the incision, foul-smelling pus began to ooze out. He ordered a biopsy culture of the exudate along with blood work.

> *Oddly enough, I felt completely comfortable and safe.*

Not surprisingly, I was once again admitted to the hospital. High doses of IV antibiotics were begun and I arrived at my room just before midnight. Oddly enough, I felt comfortable and safe. I was greeted by Patty, an RN who I had the pleasure of meeting the last time I was admitted. Was this home away from home?

Todd made sure I was settled in, placed phone calls and sent text messages to update everyone on my status.

"All's good."

He reached over and gave me a kiss good night. "Get some rest. I love you and I will talk to you in the morning."

Burton's Take

When driving I do some of my best thinking. My thoughts were Cancer has a fight on its hands to get this girl. There are so many positive vibes under Todd and Luci's roof. The feeling of concern was there but the feeling it will all work out was also there.

31

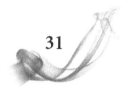

Ask and You Shall Receive

… we concur, the drainage tube needs to be removed.

I awoke around 8 a.m. I couldn't help but smile just a little—I already knew what I wanted to order for breakfast, without having to look at the menu. While I waited for my breakfast, I got dressed and freshened up. The one up side to being bald is the time needed to get one's self ready; from start to finish, 20 minutes tops. Now I could actually get myself ready more quickly than Todd.

There was a knock at my door. An older gentleman of medium build entered my room when I called out to invite whoever was there. "Hello Lucille, I am with the visiting eucharistic ministers and would like to offer you communion if you would like to receive it."

This was a nice change. Since my diagnosis and my fear of crowds, I had not been able to make it to mass. I had been confined to watching mass via the television and I missed going. All I could say, though, was, "Yes, thank you."

Shortly after, Dr Schmitz entered my room telling me that she had been notified of my call last night and reviewed all of the ER progress notes this morning. She was, as always, cheerful and upbeat when she came in to check on me. I welcomed her smile as she said, "Well, I've spoken with Dr. Hoeffer and we concur, the drainage tube needs to be removed. This will be scheduled for tomorrow."

My biggest concern was whether or not my body would be able to once again perform this function on its own without the assistance of manual draining. This was the million dollar question …

Tuesday morning I was brought down to the operating room, where I was greeted by Dr. Hoeffer. "Well, are you ready?" he asked.

"Not like I have a choice, but yes, I am ready to get rid of this tube."

"I have been in constant communication with your visiting nurse, Connie, and the fluid has been decreasing with every extraction. This is a good sign. I just hope it's not too soon."

This procedure was similar to the placement of the tube, just quicker. I once again declined general anesthetic and opted for a local block. Within 15 minutes he was done. He did caution me to expect increased sensitivity in the rib area due to the formation of scar tissue, adding that the sensitivity will decrease over time but could last for up to a year.

Todd was waiting in my room when I was brought back. We had lunch together and were later joined by Ray and Sherri. The afternoon turned out to be very pleasant for all of us.

And to think, all I really wanted for Christmas was to have the tube removed. My wish came true. I felt more freedom coming my way.

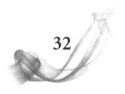

Not Again ....!

*"I think it would be best to go to the ER.
Tomorrow is Christmas Eve ..."*

What a great feeling to have the drainage tube removed. Connie was still on schedule to visit me this morning at home even though the drainage tube had been removed. Dr. Hoeffer felt it would be best to ensure the wound was healing from the inside out. Failure to keep the wound open could potentially result in a "pocket" within my body, increasing the risk of an internal infection. That was Connie's job this morning. And, with my immune system at an all time low, it was of primary importance. I was clear and accepting of the necessity, but apprehensive, nevertheless.

Around 8:30 a.m., I was feeling flushed, so once again I reached for my thermometer ... It was 99.5. "Okay, it's a slightly elevated. Try to remain calm." I tried to return to what I was doing, but I couldn't let go of this number. I took my temperature again. 99.7. My heart began to beat faster. I picked up the phone and tried to call Todd … No answer.

I was getting desperate. Today was December 23rd and I knew Ray and Sherri were planning to leave sometime this morning to go to their daughter's for Christmas. I hoped they were still there.

I felt strongly I should call them, just in case I needed a ride to the hospital. I thought I was calm, but as soon as Sherri answered, I began crying. "My temperature is rising and I can't get a hold of Todd."

"We'll be right down." Within five minutes they were "downstairs" and walked in to find me sitting, rocking in my recliner, crying. Sherri came over to console me while I blubbered out my concerns again.

Connie arrived shortly after Ray and Sherri. Ray greeted her and gave her an update. Examining my incision, she explained to me the importance of keeping the wound open. To accomplish that she would need to insert a sterile Q-tip into the opening. The potential for another painful procedure was definitely one way to get my mind off of my elevated temperature … which it did. I sat at the kitchen table and Sherri stood behind me and rubbed my shoulders while Connie prepared to "operate."

As she gently forced the Q-tip into the incision, I grabbed onto Sherri's hands and let out a horrifying scream. I can't put into words the excruciating pain of that modest action. You would have thought my liver was being ripped out. "STOP, STOP, NO MORE!!!!" Connie stopped.

> *At this point, we could have driven blind to the hospital."*

"We're almost done; I just need to pack it with a 'bleed ribbon'. This will help keep the wound open and allow healing from within." I took a deep breath, braced myself and once again held onto Sherri's hands on my shoulders, knowing now what was coming.

Just as Connie finished, Todd walked in. What a relief to see him. In an emotional rush, I told him what was going on. Echoing my concern, Connie said, "I think it would be best to go to the ER. Tomorrow is Christmas Eve. At least if you have it checked out today, there is a greater chance of your doctor being available."

So once again, Todd and I headed to the ER. At this point, we could have driven blind to the hospital.

33

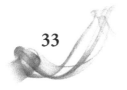

Think Twice Before You Speak

As I sat there on the bed, it suddenly occurred to me, I did not remember smelling the Heparin.

Todd and I arrived at the ER at 10:30 a.m. I was escorted to room 21 right away where Dr. Bryson met us. I gave him an overview of my history and told him I had just been released from the hospital on Tuesday following my drainage tube removal. Performing a brief exam, he ordered a blood sample of my port to rule out any infection. He also told me he wanted to speak with my oncologist prior to any other treatment. As he left the room, he told me a nurse would be in shortly to draw some blood.

Within minutes Holly entered the room. At this point in my case, I have become apprehensive—perhaps paranoid would be a better word—when it comes to my port. I couldn't help but ask her what her experience was with accessing ports and caring for cancer patients. She reassured me of her skill and ability as she began to gather the necessary items and set up a sterile surgical tray.

I took a deep breath as she penetrated the port with a Huber needle. Thankfully, the access went well, with little pain. After drawing two vials of blood she said, "Before I remove the needle, I want to check with the doctor to be sure that he only needs two vials of blood to be drawn. I'll be right back."

> *I'm sorry, but did you flush my port with Heparin?*

She returned moments later. "We're good. Dr. Bryson is just waiting on a phone call from your oncologist." As she removed the needle from my port, she added, "Once they converse, you'll be free to go." Holly cleaned up the surgical tray and then left the room.

Todd said, "This could take a while. I'm going to make a visit to the cafeteria. Would you like anything?"

"No, thanks, I'm fine."

"Okay, I'll be right back."

I sat there on the bed, it suddenly occurred to me, I did not remember smelling the Heparin. For anyone who has had a port, you know the importance of having the port flushed with Heparin after each access. This reduces the risk of blood clots forming. Heparin has a very distinct smell, not easily missed.

I started to get myself worked up when a young woman entered my room with a handful of papers. "Lucille, I have a few instructions to go over with you, and I need a signature, but then you'll be free to go …"

I quickly interjected. "Could you please get Holly for me? I have a question for her." The young woman smiled and left the room.

Holly appeared. "You have a question?"

"I'm sorry but did you flush my port with Heparin?"

She was silent for a moment and then, with hesitation, said, "You know, I didn't. I'm sorry." My heart began to beat faster and my palms started to get sweaty. I reached in my purse for my phone. "Let me call my oncologist's office and speak to Karen or Judy. I'm sure the port needs to be flushed with Heparin every time it is accessed."

Dr. Schmitz's receptionist Gail answered the phone and I explained to her where I was and what was going on. She immediately patched me through to Judy. "Yes, Luci, the port should be flushed with Heparin."

"That's what I thought." I looked over toward Holly and handed my phone to her. "You need to speak to Judy."

Holly spoke to Judy and then handed me the phone. "I'll be right back and we'll get your port flushed."

I don't know if this is true in all scenarios, but from my work with yoga and within the dental practice, I do know when one of the senses is compromised, the others become heightened. The door to my room was open. As I sat on the bed waiting, all I could see was the bathroom across from my doorway. I did remember, as a frequent "guest" to the ER, there was a nurse's station just to the right of my room. I could hear a conversation taking place in low voices. I sat very still and listened.

I heard a female's voice ask, "Do you know where we keep the Heparin flush?" I think it was Holly's.

A male voice responded, "Why?"

"Well, I just accessed a patient's port and her oncologist's nurse told me we need to flush the port with Heparin." It was Holly.

"Well then, let *her* do it."

My entire body stiffened with what I just heard—who was that asshole? I had been through so much these past three months. I tried to keep myself calm, but, the truth be told, this was my breaking point.

A few minutes later, Holly returned. It was all I could do to refrain from being hostile. I was very calm as I asked her, "Who were you talking to outside of my room?"

She replied, "I was speaking to another nurse about the Heparin."

"What is his name?" I asked, as my voice began to rise just before I completely lost it.

"Steve."

"WHO THE FUCK DOES HE THINK HE IS? THIS IS MY LIFE ON THE LINE. HOW DARE HE!"

Holly jumped toward the door to close it. She reached for the tissues and tried to calm me down. I was so angry, I was crying and shaking. "I WANT TO SEE YOUR SUPERVISOR NOW. I AM NOT LEAVING THIS ROOM."

Holly did manage to get me somewhat calmed down. She was obviously caught off guard. I know her biggest concern right now was to gain re-access to my port and properly flush it with Heparin. She was overly caring and gentle.

"Just let me flush your port first and then I will get my supervisor for you." My reaction obviously startled her. She appeared flustered but kept her composure doing the re-entry into the port. She then exited my room, closing the door partially behind her.

Darcee, the charge nurse, came in. "Holly told me what happened and I am so sorry for Steve's behavior. He's a jokester at times."

Somewhat composed, I responded, "His behavior is unacceptable." I wasn't done. Still enraged by what I had overheard, I said, "I want to see that Mother Fucker. Get him in here. I am not leaving until I can talk to him."

At that time, Todd entered the room and was shocked to see the state I was in. "WHAT'S WRONG; IS SOMETHING WRONG?" I just put up my hand and shook my head. Todd sat down in the chair at the side of my bed. Darcee left my room and shortly thereafter, a male figure entered the room and closed the door behind him.

He was mid to late 30s, about 5'8" and a husky build. My eyes were drawn to his left hand, which bore a wedding band. He said right away, "I am sorry for what I said."

I wanted to be so strong, but could not hold back the tears. "You Fucking Asshole. How dare you; this is my life that's on the line here. You obviously are in the wrong career. I hope your wife never gets cancer. Get out of my fucking sight. Get out!" The tears overflowed, my body felt exhausted.

Steve leaned up against the wall with his hands interlaced in front of him. As I proceeded to curse him out, his posture became slouched and he bowed his head down. Opening the door without a word he then left the room.

I reached for another tissue to dry my tears. As I looked over at Todd, he too began to cry.

"Let's go home."

34

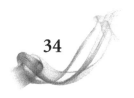

Christmas

***Just three years prior, Todd proposed to me
on this day.***

I can't say this was the best Christmas we've ever had, but I can say I was thankful to be alive and with Todd to celebrate it. Even though neither of us spoke openly of it, we couldn't help but think it. Would this be the last Christmas we share together? Just three years prior, Todd proposed to me on this day. Life, at best, offers always unexpected, unanticipated twists and turns.

We planned on spending Christmas in Utah with my family. My diagnosis changed those plans. There was no way I was about to subject my compromised immune system to any large crowds of people. Especially on an airplane; or, as I like to say—a flying, bacteria-growing, petri dish. A road trip was also ruled out. I was not physically or emotionally ready or able to embark on a nine hour journey in a car.

It felt right.

Reluctantly, we agreed it would be best to stay home and make the best of the situation at hand. It felt right.

Christmas morning, we sat in front of our little tree and opened our gifts. There weren't many, but the few we had were intimate and personal.

Todd had always wanted a PlayStation 3 (PS3). I was against this because I didn't want to lose my husband to video game after video game. But I didn't care anymore. Maybe this would give him an outlet to detach and just let go for awhile.

Todd bought me a beautiful crystal Rosary Bracelet and a ceramic Hallmark ornament, "Beautiful You." I loved them.

We spent the rest of the day, as we have done every year since we've been together, with Tara and Rafferty, our family unit curled up watching *It's A Wonderful Life a*nd *The Polar Express*.

Todd's Take

Our home had become a revolving door B&B for our family. As Luci mentioned, our home is not particularly spacious. We had my parents stay individually: Luci's Mother, Aunt Lu and Brother Jerry had come. During Pat and Frank's visit, I slept on a cot in our office for a few nights.

With Christmas approaching, Aunt Lu's illness and inability to travel was a reprieve. Don't get me wrong, I am so appreciative of all the love, support and care that our family had supplied. But, no matter how comfortable you are with your family, they are still guests. As their host, I needed to provide some company and comfort for them. I asked Luci if we could spend Christmas alone this year, I was ready to have our home to ourselves for a few days.

As it turned out, this was just what we needed. We even took a few pictures in front of the tree!

35

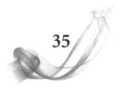

Knit One, Purl Two

My first project was going to be a hat. At this point in my life, you couldn't have too many hats.

The past three months have taken their toll on me—not just the medical issues. Suddenly removed from my busy and active, personal and professional lives has been a trial. So far, I had been doing a pretty good job keeping myself occupied though, through meditation, with my mandala coloring book, reading and watching funny movies. But I must admit, with my gradual recovery, I was beginning to get bored. I thought to myself, maybe I should learn how to knit. I definitely had the time, so why not; it couldn't be that hard.

It just so happened that Debbie and two other girls from my office were coming to visit me. I had mentioned to her my new interest, and, as I greeted them at the door, Debbie handed me a basket. The basket had balls of yarn, knitting needles, a pattern book and a beginner's step-by-step guide to knitting. I was thrilled and couldn't wait to get started. They visited with me for about three hours, catching me up on all the gossip and office goings-on, and then they headed back to Denver.

After they left, I read through the knitting guide. Maybe this was going to be more of a challenge than I had anticipated. Sherri was on my speed dial—I shared with her my new interest and wanted to know if she knew how to knit.

"Oh gosh, Luci, it's been years. Let me try to refresh myself."

My first project was going to be a hat.

The next day, she called and said she had been practicing her "cast on" technique and thought she could help me get started. "Why don't you and Todd come *upstairs* for dinner and bring your needles and yarn."

"Sounds like a plan. See you around 5 p.m."

Todd and I went *upstairs* to Ray and Sherri's around five for dinner. After eating, the guys retreated to the living room to watch TV, leaving us to our new project. We sat at the kitchen table with our needles in hand and began. It took a few tries, but when I got comfortable with the needles, I finally managed to "cast on" and start knitting.

My first project was going to be a hat. At this point in my life, you couldn't have too many hats.

My first knitted hat was complete. It was not without dropped stitches, which formed little holes throughout it—good for air circulation—but nonetheless, it resembled a hat and that was a start.

I was hooked, so to speak, on knitting. Once I got the hang of it, I found it to be quite relaxing and easy to do while watching TV. I started on my second hat, and what an improvement from the first one.

I started on my third hat. They say "Third time's the charm." This hat was perfect; no dropped stitches and it had an invisible seam! I continued on, making hat after hat. This soon became my new focus. My head was truly accessorized.

36

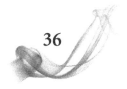

Something to Look Forward To (A Night Out)

... it had been six weeks since I had seen the doctors or my staff. I was also ready to get dressed up and have somewhere to "go out on the town."

Today, December 30th, was my 4th round of chemo. This had now become a routine for us—every third Thursday I had chemotherapy. I actually began to feel as though progress was being made. I was on the positive downward slope to completion. Two to go.

Today was similar to the prior three appointments. My white blood count was at 2.3 after having the Neulasta shot following my last treatment. I could only imagine what it would have been if I didn't have that shot. Thankfully, I was above 2.0, which was the cutoff for being able to get my treatment today. As with many, my white blood cells had been hit hard by the chemotherapy drugs. I would again return home with a Neulasta injection.

Once again Debbie from my office came to sit with me during my treatment. Having her with me while I lay in the "Chemo Room" with the IV was a Godsend. It also gave Todd a chance to meet up with his friends for coffee or lunch—a clearly needed "break" and therapy for him with the complex routine of my therapy and family visits plus keeping his business going. The worry about me; the strain of juggling all my appointments and family visits; the pressure of meeting all his commitments to his customers; and the overall upheaval in our lives was taking a toll on him—his alcohol intake was starting to increase.

While Todd spent a few hours with friends, I immersed myself with Debbie. It allowed me to stay connected with the office, and I couldn't wait to show Debbie my newest creations. "That's just like you, Luci. You set your mind to do something and you do it. You're amazing."

"Thanks Deb, not only for those kind words, but thank you for coming to sit with me. It truly means the world to me."

We spent the remainder of our time visiting about things at work and our upcoming dental practice holiday party. For six years now, our practice has had our holiday party in January. This was by chance. It all started when the restaurant where I wanted to have our party at was completely booked. Their first availability was the Saturday following New Years. Disappointed, I went ahead and booked it for the January date.

It was a big success! Everyone was more relaxed and engaging with one another. There were no worries about the upcoming holiday and the endless "to do" lists. In fact, I think having the party in January actually gave all of us something to look forward to after all the craziness the Holidays can bring. Ever since then, our holiday and end of year party for our practice is always after New Years in January.

I have always looked forward to planning it. Typically, I would start my planning for it in the heart of summertime with a notation on my August calendar, "book holiday party." This year our party was going to be at The Summit Steak House. With my appetite I was really looking forward to this. It had been six weeks since I had seen the doctors or the rest of my staff outside of Debbie. Plus, I was also ready to get dressed up and have somewhere to "go out on the town." It could be good for both Todd and I.

During my routine exam with Dr. Schmitz, the possibility of a hernia surfaced. The area just to the left of my belly button was slightly swollen and tender to pressure. In her judgment, we should keep an eye on it and wait a bit. We both felt that I was in no condition to undergo any type of surgery, due to the increased risk of infection. She also felt that the tissue around the belly button may have become weakened due to the initial surgical incision in October. Assuring me this was common and I was not at risk, I have to say it just added one more thing to worry about …

CA-125: 117! Progress!

Todd's Take

My wife was going through a fight for her life. The frequent trips to the hospital and airport wore me down, especially the trips to the ER. Trying to keep my small business afloat was a constant worry. I began to "self-medicate." What once were two or three beers after work were becoming six or eight to unwind. Sometimes it was a half-liter of Scotch to fall asleep. I don't consider myself an alcoholic although the "experts" would beg to differ. Drinking was a habit I would have to change. I just dealt with my stress as best I could at the time. I wanted to be numb.

37

MAC Attack

About a week after my fourth treatment, I noticed my eyebrows and eyelashes becoming sparse. I decided to take some action.

Up to this point, things were going as well as could be expected, but the news of a possible hernia really wore on me. I was beginning to see the effects of the chemo, both physically and emotionally. I had completely lost the hair on my head, arms, legs, underarms, private area, and my soft, fine facial hair. I also began to notice changes in my eyesight, and yes … chemo brain.

I never really gave much thought to the hair on my face. Now that it was gone, however, I realized how much it added to the fullness and completeness of my look. At least I still had my eyebrows and my eyelashes. But my face now looked very gaunt, and the pigmentation of my skin, especially my face, was very pale and pasty in color. I would be lucky to get Miss Congeniality in a beauty contest at this point.

About a week after my fourth treatment, I noticed my eyebrows and eyelashes becoming sparse. I decided to take some action. I needed something to lift my spirits. I always felt better when I took the time to do my makeup. I loved the MAC brand of makeup. In my opinion, their color palette for eye makeup compares to no other. I called the MAC location closest to me to schedule a makeup consultation. The stars were in alignment—there was an opening the following day. As I hung up the phone, a smile crossed my face; a makeover was something to look forward to.

My fear of crowds and contagion still remained, so I wanted an appointment during the week and at 10:00 a.m. when they opened. I figured this would pose the least amount of risk to me.

I was so excited. Todd dropped me off at 10, and he headed to Game Stop to check out the games for his new PS3. This MAC store was located inside Macys. I was greeted by a woman as I walked up to the consultation booth. I told her I had an appointment for a makeup consultation.

"Oh yes, you are scheduled with our makeup artist, Brandon. He will be right with you."

A young, slender male who appeared to be in his late 20s approached me. "Hi Luci, I'm Brandon and I'll be doing your makeup today."

I jumped off the chair and stepped back. "I'm sorry Brandon, but you sound like you have a cold."

"I do have a little bit of a cold."

"Did this just start or is it at the tail end?"

"It started about two days ago."

I nervously said "I'm sorry, but I can't be around anyone who is sick. This isn't going to work."

Todd quietly said, "My wife has cancer and she would like some help with her makeup."

Without saying another word, I grabbed my purse and quickly walked toward the exit. Pulling my phone out, I called Todd; there was no answer. I redialed, and again, no answer. Where the hell is he? He just dropped me off five minutes ago. I started to panic and tears began to fill my eyes. Finally after the sixth try, Todd answered. "What's up?"

"The guy who was supposed to do my makeup is sick. I can't be in here with him. Where are you? I need to get out of here and you have the keys to the car." I'm now hysterical and tears are streaming down my face.

Todd tried to calm me down. "Okay, I will be right there. Give me two minutes."

I stood in the foyer of Macy's, crying as I waited for Todd. How could this be happening, all I wanted to do was have my makeup done?

Todd pulled up in front of the doors and I got into the car. I was crying almost uncontrollably. Trying to console me, Todd asked, "Is there another MAC store in town?"

"Yeah, in the Cherry Creek Mall," I said trying to catch my breath.

"Okay then, let's go there."

"But what about all the crowds?"

In a calm, reassuring tone he said, "You have your surgical masks, don't you?"

"Yes," I replied.

"Well then, you'll just wear one of them as we walk through the mall. It's still early so it shouldn't be that crowded."

We arrived at Cherry Creek Mall just before 11. Donning my blue surgical mask, we ventured inside and walked swiftly, maneuvering our way through the mall to the MAC store. Entering my target, I took my mask off and looked for assistance.

We were quickly greeted by Rue, a young woman who was both friendly and bubbly. "So what's going on?" she said with a smile. Tears began to fill my eyes and I could not respond to her question—I was speechless, something that is alien to me.

Todd quietly said, "My wife has cancer and she would like some help with her makeup. She is really concerned with the thinning of her eyebrows and eyelashes."

If there are angels on this earth, I was standing by one. Todd has been my angel throughout, and when he spoke to Rue, I felt surrounded by wings.

Rue just smiled as she handed me a tissue. "You've come to the right place; there are plenty of options for us. Just have a seat here and I'll be right back with some color choices."

Todd just stood behind me rubbing my shoulders. Moments later, Rue returned with a large selection. As she laid them out, she said she thought it might be best to go with softer, cooler colors since my skin tone was very pale.

Rue went on to show me how to create, thicker, fuller eyebrows using a brown shadow and brow brush. She also selected a mascara that gave fullness to my lashes but was gentle and easy to remove. Todd watched Rue do her magic—I could tell by his expression she was doing a great job and could feel my shoulders relaxing.

She completed my look with a coordinating lipstick and lip gloss. Handing me a mirror, Rue asked, "Well, what do you think?"

"WOW, I love it! Thank you, Rue." The smile on my face lit up the room. Smiling back at me, "It was my pleasure. Would you like to buy any of the products I used today?"

"I will take everything."

"Oh! Okay, let me get these products together for you. I will also give you a makeup card that will show you how and where to apply the specific colors so you'll remember how to recreate this look. I'll be right back."

Rue completed my transaction and said, as she handed me the shopping bag which contained my new look, "I have written my name on your receipt. Call me any time if you have any questions about how to apply your make up."

I said, "Thank you very much; you don't know how important this was to me." I discreetly handed her a folded $20 bill and carefully replaced my surgical mask. As we left the store, I felt I had just met another angel. My grin was as broad as my mask.

Todd's Take

Luci was looking quite gaunt. She was ready for a makeover and was so looking forward to meeting with a make-up consultant. The trip to Macy's was filled with anticipation. She wanted to look good for her holiday party in January. After I dropped her at the entrance, I parked the car and went to purchase a few video games for my new game console. As the phone rang, I saw it was

Luci. I knew she was close so I didn't answer, HUGE MISTAKE; the make-up artist was sick! When I called her back, she was distraught and angry with me! This was one more hurdle she was not prepared for. Thank God, we were in Denver; there had to be another MAC store in the city. Within a few moments, we were able to locate one in Cherry Creek. It was still early so the mall would not be crowded. Off we went!

Walking through the mall, Luci's face was covered with a surgical mask. I noticed a few uncomfortable glances and I was tempted to say, "She has cancer! The mask is to keep her from inhaling your crap!"

When we got to the MAC store, Luci took a seat in the corner, away from the entrance. I went to an associate to let her know what we needed. After the incident at the ER, Rue was exactly what Luci needed: considerate, accommodating and patient, Rue restored my faith in the kindness of strangers.

38

A Set Back

***"… I am so sorry Luci, but we need to postpone
your treatment until next week."***

It was January 18th and Aunt Lucy was flying in today. Fully recovered from the flu, she had rescheduled her flight from November to January to spend the next ten days with me. With my fifth chemo treatment scheduled for Thursday, she would find that a lot had changed since she was last here at the end of October.

We arrived at Dr. Schmitz's office at 8 a.m. As with the past four treatments, Karen prepped my port for my chemo and drew my CBC. She returned shortly and I just knew something was not right. Karen was not her normal, cheerful self. Instead, a serious, disappointed tone emerged as she said, "Your platelets seem to be quite low; I'm going to draw another vial of blood."

My disappointment and concern was palpable. I had been doing so well so far; I simply had to keep on track.

The three of us just sat there quietly. Aunt Lucy clearly showed signs of nervousness.

"I just spoke with Dr. Schmitz. Because your platelets are at 40, they are too low to do chemo today. The risks are too great. I am so sorry Luci, but we need to postpone your treatment until next week." Karen's words felt like a sledge hammer had hit me.

As I packed up my belongings, Judy, the receptionist, scheduled me for the same time the following week. Handing me my new appointment card, she said, "Another one of our patients had the same thing happen to her. She swore by taking two tablespoons of Tahini every day that it helped her platelets to rebound."

I thanked her, wondering if Tahini would work for me—I was willing to try anything.

The ride home was long and quiet for three of us. Todd did make a quick stop to Natural Grocers to buy some Tahini.

I spent much of the evening alone in my room.

Following my disappointment yesterday, I was feeling emotionally weak—I was beginning to think things were taking a turn for the worse. I thought going to Mass would help lift my spirits at the church here in Bailey; they offered daily mass at 8:30 a.m. I felt my risk of exposure would be minimal, since attendance during the week was usually between seven and ten people.

A Set Back

The pastor, Father Kizzy, had come to visit me twice before at home since my surgery and he recognized us right away as we entered church. We sat in the last row of pews. During the offering of our intentions, Father Kizzy said to the congregation, "May we also pray for Luci Berardi's healing; we pray to the Lord." The congregation responded, "Lord hear our prayer." Tears filled my eyes.

After Mass, he greeted us in the vestibule. "Luci, it's so good to see you." He had a big smile on his face and reached out his arms to hug me. I told him I was upset about having my treatment delayed. "We are all praying for you. Have faith."

> *I noticed red dots on my lower legs. It looked like a bruise.*

With my treatment at a stand-still, I retreated to the Internet to research the problem of chemo and a low platelet count. I came across a blog about dark, leafy greens enhancing the increase in platelets. So I continued to eat Tahini every day and added dark, leafy greens. What harm could it do? I couldn't proceed with any treatment until my numbers increased.

I scheduled a follow-up blood draw for Monday with Conifer Medical to see if my platelets had improved. As I was getting ready for my appointment, I noticed red dots on my lower legs. It looked like a bruise. The mesh pouf

I used in the shower must have bruised my skin. This couldn't be good.

Arriving at Conifer Medical, I once again followed the protocol set by Dr. Matthews. Concerned with my risk of contracting the flu or some other sickness, he arranged for me always to be seen for a CBC check immediately upon arrival. Each time, I was to call in to the schedulers to inform them of my arrival. I would then go to the back entrance, and ring the bell where a medical lab technician would meet me. Taken directly to the lab, blood would be drawn and I would be out within five minutes.

Sheila met me this morning. As we proceeded to the lab, I saw Dr. Matthews who came over to say hello. I told him about my postponement and showed him my leg.

Looking at it he said, "It's called petechiae, and is common with patients who have low platelets. It will go away in a few days. Bruising is very common, so be very careful and try not to injure yourself. Also keep in mind, your ability to clot may also be compromised. Nose bleeds are also another common concern. You just need to give your body some time. If you have any other questions, don't hesitate to call me."

"Thank you, Dr. Matthews." I was grateful for the information and relieved.

Sheila drew a vial of blood … 37. They were still dropping.

I was still tentatively scheduled for my fifth treatment on Thursday of that week. After checking with Judy at

A Set Back

Dr. Schmitz's office, she suggested I come in on Wednesday to check my platelets once again.

They were at 48 and beginning to rise, but still too low for treatment. I really began to get worried. I asked to speak with Dr. Schmitz if she was available.

"Of course, let me go and get her for you." Judy left the room. Todd and I sat and waited.

Dr. Schmitz came in. As always she had a smile on her face and was very empathetic to my plight: I was quite concerned the prognosis was going to be compromised with these delays.

She did her best to reassure me. "In accordance with the American Cancer Society, a patient may delay treatment up to three weeks without negatively affecting the long-term outcome."

From the beginning, she has always been up front and honest with me. I had no reason not to believe this, but somehow I just couldn't wrap my head around this one … Paranoia once again was rearing its ugly head. My treatment was delayed yet another week. To make matters worse, Aunt Lucy was leaving tomorrow.

Todd's Take

The news that Luci could not get her chemo treatment was a huge cloud overhead. We both knew she was taking the maximum dose. It was evident that the chemo was doing something, I tried to console her and validate that this was actually a good thing. Luci's CA-125 was dropping; the cancer was dying. The chemo on the other hand had reduced her ability to fight off any illness which could kill her. Her body just needed some time to recover from the poison that was being put into her. The doctors told us this was normal.

To Luci, this was a set-back. It meant that she was prolonging the treatment and her ability to get back to living normally. In her mind, a lull in scheduled treatment was giving the cancer an opportunity to re-grow. I know it scared the hell out of her. I did my best to console her; we had to trust the doctors.

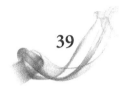

My Darkest Hour

For the first time since my diagnosis, I actually thought I may not win this fight.

I knew deep down in my heart the chemo was working on the cancer, by the C-125 results … But was it also working against my other internal organs and body functions?

Was it working against my mind as well? It began to affect me emotionally. How could Todd possibly love "this?" I was so thin, bald and pale. *I was ugly.* There was no getting around it.

While the chemo was winning, my body was losing the fight. I could feel I was losing control of my thoughts and being sucked down into a depressive state of mind. For the first time since my diagnosis, I actually thought I may

> *You need to remember all the things that you are grateful for.*

not win this fight. Briefly—just for the proverbial split second—I questioned myself.

"What's the point? I'm going to die."

What I couldn't bear was to leave this visual image of myself in the minds of Todd and my family and friends. Thank God for ego, and—by the grace of God—somewhere deep within me, I knew enough to call Rita, my best—my closest—friend, who knows me better than I know myself.

I can honestly say, I have never felt such helplessness in my life. Once again Rita talked me through this funk I had fallen in.

"You need to remember all the things you are grateful for. You are alive; you are surrounded by so many people who care about you and love you; and your blood marker has been dropping at record percentages!"

In silence, I absorbed her words. Then she continued. "Your body is fighting like it has never fought before. It may just need a break from those chemicals. Don't give up."

She also suggested trying a writing technique which she has found to be very helpful. "Luci, I want you to get a pad of paper and begin writing what it is you desire."

We spent an hour on the phone together … and I was beginning to feel better. Just connecting, hearing her voice was soothing. Rita always had a practical, common sense side to her. At the same time, her genuine warmth flowed through the phone lines.

"Luci you know I am always here for you, and if you need me to come there right now I will; just say the word."

"No Ri, that's not necessary, I actually do feel much better having talked through this with you. Thank you."

"Okay, but just say the word ... I will talk with you tomorrow, okay?"

"Yeah."

"Love you 'Cille."

"Love you too, Ri."

I began writing:

> My intent is to have my platelets increase naturally when my body is ready. I am in control of my thoughts. You are cancer, you will not win this battle. My body will heal itself in its own time. *Fuck You, Cancer!*

I continued to re-write this. Over and over again I wrote, until I had filled two pages. Then I set my notepad down, said The Healing Prayer and the prayer to St. Peregrine and went to bed.

Aunt Lu's Take

The days and nights that followed were very depressing and seemed very dark and long. Luci would sit in the recliner trying to keep busy—reading, knitting, etc. But I knew she was ready to jump out of her skin. Her legs started to shake and she was crying on the phone with her best friend Rita.

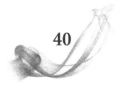

40

Something to Look Forward to

One thing that helped me keep emotionally on track was being able to have something to look forward to.

With each day, my emotional state had begun to improve. Some days were harder than others, but I was determined to keep my mind focused on the positive and dismiss the negative mind chatter as soon as it started. This, however, was sometimes harder than fighting the disease itself …

One thing that helped me keep emotionally on track was being able to have something to look forward to. Faced with a true life-threatening event, one's mind can become consumed with regretful thoughts. "If only I had done…," or, "I wish had …"

I did regret not visiting Utah more. I wished I had as many adult memories with my family as I did when I was a child. With that, I resurrected the idea of how great it would be to go on a trip now with my brothers and our spouses.

I felt like a new woman ...

Why not a cruise? I have always wanted to go on a cruise to Alaska. I've only heard wonderful things about cruising to Alaska. Just for a Moment, I hesitated. What if the cancer isn't gone, or what if it comes back? What about all those people on the cruise ship—I could catch something.

Yes, and there was a possibility I could still be in treatment. But there was also a possibility that I could get in a car accident on my way to a doctor's appointment and die as well. We don't know—can't know—the future. It's easy to become paralyzed and live in fear of "what if …?" I was not going to give away my power and let this disease control me. That's why there's travelers insurance!

I called Frank and Jerry to see what they thought of this idea. They both agreed. It was a great idea. We also all agreed that July would be the best month. I told them I would start researching the cruise lines and their schedules. Frank and his wife, Tiff, have cruised several times and had really good luck with Cruise One Travel Agency. I contacted Tammy at Cruise One and she helped me with all the arrangements.

Todd was elated. I was talking and planning for a future event. We chose a mini-suite with a balcony. As far as I was concerned, you only live once …

Everything was set.

Even though the cruise wasn't for seven months, the excitement and anticipation for the cruise gave me something to focus my attention toward. In fact, I didn't stop there. I planned a long weekend trip to Utah in April to see my family, especially my niece and nephew, Brooklyn and Braxton. With the exception of Mom and Aunt Lucy's visits and the one visit by Jerry in October and Frank in December, I hadn't seen anyone since October. The month of May would be a great time to go back home to Topeka, Kansas, to see Todd's family. We set aside the Memorial Day weekend. And last but not least, we wanted to go back to New York. Todd had only been there once before, in 2009. I booked our tickets and room reservation for the first week in June. And once again, bought travelers insurance. There was no worry of remorse … only excitement for our upcoming vacations.

I felt like a new woman.

Todd's Take

When Luci asked me about scheduling a cruise in July, I thought it would be a great idea. It could be a celebration of life. It also gave her something else to focus on. One thing Luci loves to do is plan, whenever we thought of a vacation spot, Luci was on line researching flights, evaluating hotels and rental car companies, always finding the best deals. One thing led to another and she soon had scheduled "Luci's Victory Tour." It was to be Utah, Kansas, New York, Alaska, British Columbia and Washington State. I was happy to oblige, I could see she was looking forward and not letting this get the best of her. Things were beginning to get back to normal.

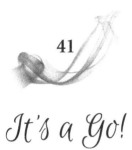

41

It's a Go!

***Let's go ahead and get you ready for your
fifth treatment."***

Todd and I arrived at Dr. Schmitz's office at 8 a.m. Today was February 3rd. Karen greeted us, smiling and as cheerful as ever. "I have a good feeling about your numbers today, Luci." She drew a vial of blood and left the room. She returned within five minutes grinning from ear to ear. "Your platelets are at 177! That's wonderful. Let's go ahead and get you ready for your fifth treatment."

I let out a sigh of relief. Simultaneously, Todd and I reached for our phones. I said, "You call your Mom and dad, and I will call my Mom and Rita."

"Got it."

Todd again had errands to run, so I sat by myself today. All I cared about was getting my chemo. I spent much of my time listening to my *Healing Bowls* CD while I brought myself into a deep, meditative, prayerful state of mind.

I was back on schedule. Todd returned around noon with lunch. We sat together and ate. The treatment concluded around 2 p.m. My next stop was to see Bob for a Reiki session. I had rescheduled my treatment from last week to today. I was really looking forward to seeing him.

CA-125 … 58!

One more treatment to go …

Todd's Take

The last few weeks had been rough on us both. Skipping one treatment was a minor setback—two was disturbing. Dr. Schmitz had told us there was a possibility that Luci would skip a few treatments. If she missed three weeks, it could allow the Cancer a toehold. We both were on edge until her numbers came back. I was so relieved when the platelet count was up.

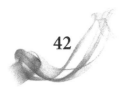

Renewed Hope

It was gratifying that she was currently cancer-free, which gave me further hope.

I decided to participate in a second cancer support group meeting. This time, however, it was conducted via a teleconference network. Participating in the support group from the comfort of my home definitely had its benefits. There were eight of us on the call. Susan, the facilitator, welcomed each of us and explained the format of the meeting. We each would introduce ourselves, explain our diagnosis, the proposed treatment, and where we were currently in the regimen.

We listened to the others, waiting our turn. One woman's story in particular caught my attention. Her name was Kate. Diagnosed a year prior to me at Stage IV, she was also BRCA I positive. It was gratifying that she was currently cancer-free which gave me further hope. What intrigued me the most was what she was actively doing to prevent a future recurrence. She was working with a naturopath, Dr. Nasha Winters, who was also an ovarian cancer survivor of 20 years. Kate briefly touched upon her diet and her current prophylactic therapy of IV Vitamin C.

> *MaMa is different ...*

When the conference call ended, I couldn't wait to tell Todd all about it. This is just what I had been searching for. It just made sense to me. There has to be a correlation between diet and cancer. I couldn't let this go. I sent an email to the facilitator, Susan, and asked if she would contact Kate. Would she be willing to speak with me, one-on-one?

Susan emailed me with Kate's email address and phone number and I sent an email to her to which she immediately responded. I was so curious to know everything Kate was doing. Kate graciously shared with me Dr. Winter's Treatment Plan for her. Her plan addressed glycemia, hormones, stress and inflammation, and blood supply. The goal is to shift her biochemistry to one that is hostile to cancer.

> *Glucose:* Cancer is glutton for glucose.
> A low glycemic diet is a must.

Hormones: Even if the tumor is negative to estrogen receptors and progesterone receptors, research shows exogenous estrogens STILL need to be avoided.

Stress: Often times stress is the biggest factor for patients. If you don't handle your stress, you won't do well. Meditation, yoga and exercise need to be implemented.

Inflammation: Inflammation promotes all kinds of growth factors. Monitor internal inflammation state.

Blood Supply: The goal is to keep blood thin/flowing as well as keeping blood supplies away from tumors. Melatonin and Vitamin C works well.

We continued to communicate back and forth through emails and occasional phone calls; and the rest is history. Although we have yet to meet, I call her my friend.

With just one more treatment to go, I felt I needed to incorporate some physical exercise. I was determined to get my pre-cancer body back along with my pre-cancer hair. I returned to my mat and began to practice gentle yoga at home. In addition to yoga, I thought the guidance of a physical therapist might be in my best interest. Contacting my health insurance, I was relieved to find I was eligible for physical therapy coverage. All I needed was a request from Dr. Schmitz indicating the medical necessity.

Securing her support, I began physical therapy three times a week. I was truly amazed how weak and atrophied my muscles had become in such a relatively short period of time—in just a matter of months.

Rafferty's Take

MaMa is different. I feel it in her voice and see it in how she moves now. She talks to me differently—like she's happy to see me.

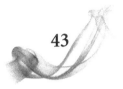

43

Chasing Rainbows

"Yeah, yeah, I am ... Because I have nothing to lose, but everything to gain ..."

I began to seriously think about going to Durango to see Dr. Winters as her recommendations seemed to be helping Kate. I sent an email to introduce myself and to ask if she would accept me as a patient. Mona, her practice manager, responded and said Dr. Winters would consider this if I would agree to come to Durango and stay for a month. A month is a long time and Durango is on the other side of the state. I thanked her for the call and told her I needed to speak with my husband.

This did not go over very well with Todd. "You haven't even completed your final chemotherapy. I think you need to wait until after you have your post-treatment CT scan

> *There was something to it; these were not just coincidences ...*

before you make such drastic decisions."

That did it—Todd made sense. I was only a few weeks away from completing the sixth chemo session. I called Mona back to inform her of my decision. She added, "Nasha feels it's best for you to work with someone in your area. She has tried unsuccessfully in the past to handle long distance doctoring and it is frustrating. Not to mention, it can be unsafe for both parties."

This was just a minor setback. I continued to spend much of my time searching for information on diet and cancer. I ordered two books from Amazon; *Anti Cancer, A New Way of Life*, written by David Servan-Schreiber, MD, PhD; and *The China Study* written by T. Colin Campbell, PhD and Thomas M. Campbell, MD. Arriving within days, I found both books to be filled with amazing information and hope. From this day forward, I began to follow the diet recommendations outlined—I may not be conferring with Dr. Winters, but I did have the words and advice that paralleled her work in these books.

My next mission was to locate a naturopath in the Denver area where I too could begin IV Vitamin C therapy, following the lead from Kate and the research I did online. (The authors of the above books did not mention vitamin C therapy.)

As I was watching the Dr. Oz show, there was a preview

for the next day's guest, Dr. Issam Nemeh. He is a former anesthesiologist who has become an acupuncturist and a faith healer. Thousands flock to have him pray over them, hoping to receive a miraculous healing of incurable conditions ranging from multiple sclerosis to paralysis to cancer.

Finally, for the first time since my diagnosis, I was being exposed to so many different potential opportunities. There was something to it; these were not just coincidences …

I couldn't wait to tell Todd about this and asked him to tape this show, because I wanted him to be able to see it too, after I had watched it.

I watched the episode. Hope was once again renewed. While I waited for Todd to return home from work, I visited Dr. Nemeh's website to see if he had any healing services scheduled in Colorado. The closest place was Phoenix, Arizona. This could be a real possibility.

When Todd came home, I couldn't wait to watch the episode again. He didn't say too much at first. I told him I went to Dr. Nemeh's website and he was going to be in Phoenix in April. Todd rubbed his face with his hands, brought his hands over the top of his head and clasped his neck.

... You are making me a little crazy with all of this.

He just sighed. "I understand you want to do everything you can to keep the cancer from coming back, but I have to tell you, you are making me a little crazy with all of this."

I sat there quietly as Todd continued. "You're here; then you're over here; *then* you're over there … It's like you're chasing rainbows."

Tears began to fill my eyes as I responded.

"Yeah, yeah, I am … Because I have nothing to lose, but everything to gain …"

Todd's Take

Being on the positive down slope of the chemo treatments, Luci could not get enough information about cancer symptoms, treatments and prevention. The good news is that there is a lot of good information out there. The bad news is that there is a lot of information out there … treatments, therapies, healers and dietary regiments. It was all-consuming to her. It was becoming too much for me.

We had a life before the diagnosis. I wanted it back. We used to talk about work, upcoming trips, friends and family. Now, every conversation was about someone who was in their third or fourth treatment or someone who had just been diagnosed. Oprah and Dr. Oz had an episode on survivors, faith healers and prevention. Every conversation we had was about cancer.

Luci heard of a doctor in the Ohio area who had the gift of healing after watching an episode of Dr. Oz. She wanted to fly to Phoenix to meet with him. Then she was ready to jump on a plane immediately after her last treatment to go to Durango for a month. The woman I married who was always so in control was losing it. It might have been due to what is called Chemo Brain: the inability to concentrate for extended periods.

It was beginning to wear on me. After the "Chasing Rainbows" comment, we sat down and talked about it. I had to be pragmatic. My position was that Luci complete her final chemo treatment and the final scan to verify the cancer was gone. It was only three more weeks. If there was still evidence of cancer after the scan, then we should look into the other therapies. I think this made sense to her after she realized she was nearing the end of the treatment regimen. We had to trust Dr. Schmitz.

44

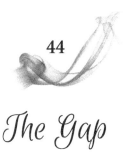

The Gap

... I was terrified. Could our marriage withstand these trials before us?

I can't speak to other events or challenges that couples face, but I can tell you these past four months have been filled with stress, anger, fear, sadness, and uncertainty. And our relationship was beginning to show it. Todd and I had only been married for two years and I was terrified. Could our marriage withstand these trials before us?

When illness enters the picture, it can splinter a relationship. The experience and outcome for couples can vary, and gender plays a role. In an article by Tara Parker-Pope, published in the *New York Times*, November, 2009:

The Gap

When the man became seriously ill, only 3 percent experienced the end of a marriage. But among women diagnosed, about 21 percent ended up separated or divorced. Among couples who split up, divorce occurred, on average, about six months after the diagnosis, although there was wide variability in the timing.

(See Tara Parker-Pope in the Notes for the link to her *New York Times* article.)

For me, going through surgery and chemotherapy directly affected my self-confidence. I had lost my femininity and my sex appeal. Living within my body for the past four months hasn't eliminated the shock I saw in the morning. A gaunt, pale and bald image looking back at me—sexy it wasn't. In addition to all of this, I was now in menopause. My night sweats made it difficult for us to cuddle with one another; and I was on an emotional rollercoaster. And because of this, I could see Todd keeping things to himself and becoming withdrawn.

Prior to becoming a couple, Todd and I had both previously sought professional counseling. As our relationship became more serious, we both felt it was important to have a complete understanding of each other's view on commitment, finances and communication. Before we got married, we felt it would be in our best interest to meet with a "couple's counselor." Now, being faced with these unexpected challenges, I am so glad we did.

The intimacy we once shared together was beginning to fade. I never once questioned Todd's commitment or love for me, but I feared if we just ignored this "elephant in the room," this little gap would only grow bigger. I too was committed to my marriage, and I refused to just let it fix itself. I was willing to do whatever it took to once again regain our intimacy.

On a Saturday, the elephant took center stage. We both openly agreed we had a problem—at least the barrier had not grown that high—but neither one of us knew what to do to correct it. We needed professional assistance. I placed a call to our therapist, Leslie. Giving her a quick overview of the recent events, I told her we needed to see her. That afternoon, she called back. She was shocked to hear our news and extended her support. She was able to see us right away.

> "... The bottom line is trust."

We talked with Leslie about the many different concerns we had. The lack of intimacy, the emotional roller coaster, the uncertainty of my long-term diagnosis, the financial uncertainty and the way in which each of us was dealing with these issues.

Leslie started by saying, "You need to have trust with one another and believe each of you is truly committed to upholding the vows you exchanged two years ago. You can't dwell on whether one of you is going to leave; that would be counterproductive. *The bottom line is trust.*"

The Gap

"Additionally, the two of you have been through a very traumatic event. There are real fears the two of you have, and only time will allow those fears to go away. As you have more and more clear scans, you will be able to let some of your walls down. You both need to think back to the time when you were dating and try to recapture those feelings and desire. It doesn't just need to be through the physical act of sex. Try holding hands; kissing each other in the morning and before going to bed; when watching TV, sit next to one another on the couch. Eat dinner together without any other interruptions; and make sure you plan date nights. You need to date all over again. You both need to look toward the future and continue living your lives together. Planning a trip is a wonderful idea because it gives you something to look forward to."

Todd and I both felt a sense of relief after our session with her. We finally had a safe place to voice our fears to one another without worrying if we were going to hurt the other person's feelings. I can't stress enough how much we needed this intervention.

Todd and I both made extra efforts to incorporate Leslie's suggestions ... Todd and I physically connected. This was the first time since before my diagnosis. We were both nervous. We didn't know what to expect. Was it going to be painful or would it feel different? We were like two teenagers having sex for the first time. Afterwards, we both had a sense of relief. This was yet another step bringing us closer together.

There was one noticeable change however, which I presume was directly related to my hysterectomy; the increase in vaginal dryness and need of lubrication assistance. All was good, until I developed a urinary tract infection two days later!

I was not too concerned about this, because Dr. Schmitz did say this is fairly common; it was because of dryness, friction and the thinner vaginal tissue. Todd however, was clearly freaked out about it.

This was, fortunately, a minor setback; overall, things were improving. We have come so far and I only had one more treatment to go. I truly believed our relationship could continue to mend itself; we just needed to get through this and my post-treatment CT scan.

A new beginning had begun …

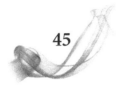

45

The Waiting Game

***Whew! What I didn't want was another visit
to the ER—I wanted it to be over!***

It was finally here; my last chemo treatment. I was so ready. I felt a huge sense of accomplishment, and rightfully so. These past five months were by far the most challenging months in my life.

Debbie once again graciously came to sit with me during my final treatment. I was given a bouquet of flowers congratulating me on my completion of treatment. My CA-125 was 24, a huge drop from the 4,472 marker just five months ago. I was hopeful that in three weeks time, my levels would indeed be within the normal range.

The next three weeks were anything but quiet. Following my final treatment, I experienced pain like I had never experienced before. Saturday evening around 11 p.m.,

I was awakened by severe pains in my stomach. The pain would come and go similar to a contraction. My first thought was, "Oh my God, the chemo now affected my organs and they were beginning to fail me."

I didn't want to alarm Todd, so I suffered through the pain. I did manage to fall back to sleep, but once again, I was awakened by intense pain in my stomach. It was 7 a.m. and I rolled over to tell Todd what was happening.

Getting me a hot compress to lay over my stomach, he asked, "Do you want me to call Dr. Schmitz?"

"Let's just wait until 8 a.m. to see if it subsides."

During this time, Todd ran down to the corner store and bought me some ginger ale. When he returned, I asked him to call Dr. Schmitz. The answering service picked up the call. Dr. Schmitz was out of town and Dr. Davis was taking calls. Explaining to Dr. Davis my symptoms, he was told that they were most likely a side effect of the chemotherapy. "Had I had any of these symptoms following any other treatments?"

"No," Todd responded.

"Well, that is very good. She's been very lucky."

Then he suggested giving me fluids and trying to see if I could tolerate some saltines. He also told Todd if things did not change by early afternoon, he should bring me to the ER. I was able to keep the ginger ale and saltines down and by 11 a.m. the pain was gone. Just like that. Whew! What I didn't want was another visit to the ER—I wanted it to be over!

I had already scheduled my CT scan for March 14th. My Mom wanted to be here for this scan so she was scheduled to arrive on the 13th.

> *The technician told me I should expect to hear from my doctor sometime tomorrow.*

I reflected back to one of Rita's conversations with me about writing out my intention. I began writing "My scan is clear" and kept praying for just that … a clear scan.

Today was the day, Todd, my Mom and I arrived at Invision Sally Jobe in Denver at 8 a.m. After an evening of fasting, I was required to drink a contrast one hour prior to my CT scan. At 9 a.m. I was brought back to change into a gown and get prepped for my scan. In addition to drinking the contrast, an IV was started to inject some type of dye. The scan was done within ten minutes. The technician told me I should expect to hear from my doctor sometime tomorrow.

I was a nervous wreck for the remainder of the day. I did what I did best to distract myself; I went into our home office and surfed the web. At 5:30 p.m., the phone rang. I could see the caller ID; it was Dr. Schmitz's office. My heart started to beat faster.

"Hello, this is Luci."

"Lucille, this is Nancy, one of Dr. Schmitz's nurses. We received your CT scan and Dr. Schmitz would like to set up an appointment to go over the results."

Oh no! Something's wrong, I thought. Then I asked, "Nancy, could you tell me what the scan showed?"

She began to read through the report. "All of the metastases in the pelvic, abdomen and lymphs were resolved. No evidence of cancer remained." I began to cry.

"When can I come in to meet with Dr. Schmitz?"

"I have an appointment open tomorrow at 2 p.m—this is good news," Nancy said, trying to offer reassurance.

"Yes, I know, I'm crying because I am happy."

"We will see you tomorrow. Thank you."

I got up from my computer and went downstairs. My Mom and Todd stopped in mid-sentence and looked toward me. "It's clear."

My Mom jumped up out of her chair and came over to the stairs "OH THANK GOD." She wrapped her arms around me, squeezed me and began crying with me. Mom then quickly let go of me and said with a smile, "Oh Todd, I'm so sorry."

Todd's eyes were filled with tears as well. He and I embraced as he whispered, "You did it!"

Mom immediately grabbed the phone to tell everyone the news. Todd also reached for his cell phone to call his parents. I returned upstairs to my bedroom. I knelt down at the side of my bed, reached for my rosary, kissed them and brought them into my heart center. I began to cry silently and just kept saying, "Thank you for hearing my prayers and healing me."

Todd's Take

The sense of relief was overwhelming. Luci had kicked this cancer in the ass. I was so happy. I knew this was going to have a profound effect on our lives. By no means has our life gone back to the pre-diagnosis normality. Luci was determined to keep the disease from taking hold again. She visited with nutritionists, naturopaths and anyone who could expand her understanding of how to keep the cancer at bay. The more she learned, the more she was determined to tell her story. Shortly after her "Clear" scan, Luci started talking about the possibility of writing a book to raise awareness and get the word out that this cancer could be beaten.

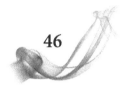

46

New Beginnings

I was still experiencing some fatigue, but each day was better than the day before.

I was now ready to try to put our lives back together—ready to return to normalcy. Todd and I knew our lives have and will forever be changed by this experience. We would now have a new "normal."

Even though I lost my hair, hair was sparsely re-growing even after I shaved my head in December. Yes, ladies, I am the bearer of bad news ... chemotherapy can kill a lot things, but even chemotherapy couldn't kill those unruly, wiry, gray hairs!!

I couldn't believe it, my gray hairs were unaffected by all that chemo. Now that my chemotherapy was complete, I was not about to give these gray hairs any advantage over my dark brown hair. On March 18th, I had Todd shave my head one last time. I wanted to start with a clean, clear slate.

I was now five weeks from my last chemotherapy. Color was beginning to return to my face, and I noticed my soft, delicate, fine facial hair coming back. Now that my chemo treatment was completed, I thought it would be worth another visit to MAC. I wanted to see if there was a possibility of wearing false eyelashes. Both the eyelashes and eyebrows had disappeared at the end of January.

Although Rue was not there on the day I went in, my experience with Monica was equally wonderful. She recommended additional colors to add to my existing palette to help create a more dramatic look, now that my pigmentation had returned.

And she also showed me how to adhere false eyelashes. Not having worn them before, I did not realize how easy it was to put them on. The key is in the application of the glue. You don't apply the glue directly to the eyelashes. Instead, you place a drop of glue on a smooth surface (the eyelashes case works well) and gently run the edge of the eyelash through the drop of glue. This gives an even distribution of the glue. Then you place the eyelashes at the lash line and gently secure them in place with a Q-tip or a toothpick. Once dried, the glue is clear and will be invisible. Not in a thousand years would I have ever guessed that I would become a false eyelash expert!

With each day came new changes. On April 3rd, six weeks post-chemotherapy, there it was … A "five o'clock shadow" of my eyebrows. They were coming back!! I also noticed tiny signs of new eyelashes. It wouldn't be long now …

I continued with physical therapy and therapeutic yoga through the end of March, and in April, I began teaching yoga again. Exercise has also become a very important component of my new lifestyle. In addition to yoga, I felt it was important to incorporate weight training. My concern was my age. I was entering into Menopause and was unable to take any medication to assist with this change.

I returned to work three days a week. I was still experiencing some fatigue, but each day was better than the day before.

Sue's Take

Luci is now back in balance, positive and can share her experience helping teach others that this illness can change you for the better. Cancer can be your greatest gift, you grow as a person, learn to value life, blessings to all. Ask God, ask Christ, they will be there for you. Fear makes us say and do that which we would not normally say or do. We must not let fear take control, but to take control and take charge of what is best for us.

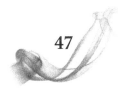

47

A Lifestyle Change

The blinding revelation: *The way I was living my life obviously was conducive to the development of cancer*

Six months following my diagnosis, I volunteered at Swedish Medical Center with The Colorado Ovarian Cancer Alliance (COCA) for the 9 News Health Fair. There I ran into Dr. Pinzinski, the hospitalist whose care I was under during my initial admission in October, 2010. Nervous at first, I was hesitant to approach him, but I wanted to let him know I was cancer-free.

I walked up to him and said, "Dr. Pinzinski, I don't know if you will remember me, but I'm Luci Berardi. I was admitted into the hospital last October with stage IV Ovarian Cancer."

He thought for a Moment and then replied, "Oh yes, I do remember you. How are you doing?"

"I am here volunteering with COCA. I am cancer-free."

"That's wonderful. You look great. I must tell you, you had a very bad diagnosis. I remember talking with my wife, who is also a physician, about your case and I was hoping you would make it to Christmas. I am so happy for you and wish you continued health."

Our conversation had a two-fold effect on me: one of shock and one of triumph. I was shocked to hear how sick I really was, but equally, I felt a sense of triumph like never before. I was truly thankful that he had not shared his medical opinion with me in October.

While mainstream medicine tries to do its best in diagnosing and treating patients, there always remains an unknown component. As the old saying goes, "Opinions are like belly buttons, we all have one." With all due respect, a doctor's opinion is just that: an opinion. They are not gods.

As a patient, I understand why some may ask their doctors, "Am I going to be okay?" Or, "How long do I have?" We ask these questions because deep down, we want the doctor to say, "Oh, you'll be fine," or, "You'll beat this." I've been there. The danger, however, is whether or not you will be ready to hear what it is they may say … For me, I didn't want to know. We had already done some reading via the Internet—we knew that ovarian cancer, especially stage IV, was not optimistic. But I didn't want that info—that news—driven in.

If I had been told I only had two months to live, perhaps my outcome may have been different. This is why I told Todd, prior to going into surgery, not to tell me any more bad news. I did not want to hear it. This just reconfirms the importance of having a positive mind-set as we enter our fight against cancer.

I can honestly say that without conventional Western Medicine, I would not be writing this book. I equally believe in the efficacy of Eastern Medicine. When you are faced with losing your life, I feel you need to be completely open to all possible therapies.

My chemotherapy was completed; I was cancer-free, and I was told to live my life. Okay, that sounded great, but how exactly was I supposed to do that? The blinding revelation: *The way I was living my life obviously was conducive to the development of cancer!*

Yes, I do have a genetic disposition, but something I was doing—or not doing—allowed the cancer to express itself. In addition to the follow-up care with my oncologist, I believed I needed the guidance of a nutritionist and a naturopath.

I also started to search for a naturopath in the Denver area who offered IV vitamin C therapy. I was directed to an integrative clinic in Boulder, Colorado. I read through their website and became intrigued with their clinic and the therapies available and requested an appointment by

> Whole Foods is a wonderful resource. Not only for their large variety of wholesome and healthy food choices, but many Whole Foods stores have a licensed nutritionist on staff. In most cases, your first 30 minute consultation is free. You may schedule future meetings for a nominal fee. I received a great deal of information from Tracy, my nutritionist. Today, many of my food choices follow the "ANDI score." ANDI stands for *Aggregate Nutrient Density Index*. ANDI scores are calculated by evaluating an extensive range of micronutrients, including but not limited to: vitamins, minerals, phytochemicals and antioxidant capacities.

email. The next day, I received a phone call from Dr. Stephen Parcell, one of the naturopaths. I gave him my brief health history. He told me I would be a great candidate for IV vitamin C therapy. We set up a "new patient consultation" appointment on March 23rd.

At my follow-up appointment with Dr. Schmitz, I told her I was seeking the assistance of a naturopath who could provide IV vitamin C therapy. She was open and receptive to my choices and gladly consented to send my records to Dr. Parcell for my upcoming appointment.

Todd and Rita both went with me to Naturemed Clinic to meet with Dr. Parcell. My first appointment was thorough and informative. The three of us felt comfortable with the information and knowledge shared by him. He went over his recommendations for supplements with us. In addition to the current vitamins, I also left with several other supplements. My IV therapy would begin next week and I would continue with a weekly treatment plan.

Still in the back of my mind was Dr. Nemeh and going to Phoenix to see him. Yes, I was given a clean bill of health, but what harm could this do? As I have mentioned several times before, I do not believe in coincidences. Here is just one more confirmation of that belief. The appearance of Dr. Nemeh, who I had recently heard of as a healer, at this time and in the nearby state of Arizona, didn't seem accidental.

After I received the miraculous news of being cancer-free, Mom, who was visiting, and I went to mass the following morning. As we sat in our pew, my eyes spied a lavender flyer in the pew pocket and I reached for it. I was stunned! "Join us on March 31st at Presentation of Our Lady Catholic Church, Denver CO, to receive a healing from Alan Ames."

Alan Ames has the gift of healing. (See Alan Ames in the Notes for his website.) Ever since 1994, Alan has been traveling to all continents to share how God lifted him from misery and hopelessness into a life full of joy and freedom. As I said, he has the gift of healing and after his talks, he prays over each of those present (by the laying on of hands). Alan's ministry enjoys the explicit permission and support of his archbishop Barry Hickey of the Catholic Diocese of Perth, Australia.

Well, my decision was now easy.

Luci's Take

Well, it was clear, I had options—and a variety of people were now crossing my path. Doors were opening—I could close them or go through them. My decision was indeed, easy.

Mom's Take

It has almost been two years now and every scan has been negative. Hopefully God has answered all our prayers and is taking Luci in his embrace.

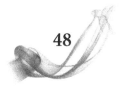

A Personal Commitment

I would like to ask you to take a Moment to really think about what I am about to ask. I encourage you get a notepad and a pen to write down your responses. "What are the things that bring you joy and happiness in your life?"

Look over your list. The things you have written down should be the reasons why you choose to make a lifestyle change. Don't think of it as being deprived or missing out on something. I think there is too much hype on the relationship between food and emotion, for example:

> I am so stressed out; I need some chocolate to help me get through this!

Really? Sound familiar? Remember my story at the beginning of this book—I could start my day inhaling chocolate! If that is one of your mantras, I truly believe you just haven't found your motivation yet. Until now, that is …

For me personally, being diagnosed with cancer and facing death was all the motivation I needed. What a wake-up call! I feel I have been given a second chance at life. Spring is a time of new life and new blossoms. Surviving this ordeal, I thought of myself as a flower that is getting ready to bloom with new life. There are too many things this flower still wants to do and see.

I believe people fail over and over again trying to lose weight, or to stop smoking, or changing to more healthy eating habits … They fail because they have the wrong focus. Most people's minds dwell on—associate with—negative thoughts. For example, when someone has a heart attack, their physician may scold them:

> You need to lose weight; you need to exercise more; you need to stop eating fatty foods; because if you don't, you're going to die.
>
> You need to … You need to … You need to.

Some patients may start out with a good intention. They will give 110 percent following their doctor's advice … at least for a short time. But they're doing it for the wrong reason.

> I need to do this (or that), because if I don't, I'm gonna die.

After a period of time you and I both know what happens:

I've been working so hard; I deserve this doughnut.

The mind begins to rationalize why it's okay to eat the doughnut. And, before you know it, they're back eating the way they did before their heart attack. Death is a huge fear; it is a negative thought. The mind doesn't want to live in fear, so it will find a way to bring joy even if it's only temporary.

Could there possibly be another way to go about this? What if the same patient was asked the question I just asked you? Perhaps her or his response may have been spending time with their children or grandchildren, traveling to foreign places, walking their dog, golfing or skiing. So now when the patient sees that doughnut, their impulse may be different. Her next thought could easily be … but if I eat that doughnut, it just may prevent me from that cruise I wanted or that round of golf.

Eating Habits

Some things are out of our control when it comes to cancer. We do, however, have absolute control over what we choose to put into our bodies and how we choose to take care of the "temple of our souls"—our physical body. It is my whole-hearted belief that making such changes to my own eating habits and my exercise routine can have a dramatic affect on reducing—possibly even preventing—a recurrence. This is why I am committed to following a very rigid meal plan.

I don't refer to the way in which I eat as a "diet." This word has a negative connotation. Saying, instead, my "eating habits" or my "eating choices," has become my preference. Many of the recommendations found in *Anti Cancer, A New Way of Life*, by Dr. David Servan-Schreiber, and *The Anti-Cancer Food and Supplement Guide*, by Debora Yost, are closely followed to maintain my new life and health.

It's not uncommon for cancer survivors to alter their eating habits and follow a vegan's lifestyle, as I did. However, I was introduced by my friend Kate, to the importance of animal protein for specific blood types and the benefits for long-term survival.

I furthered my research on specific eating recommendations based on one's blood type. *Eat Right For Your Type*, by Dr. Peter J. D'Adamo, provides very detailed dietary recommendations by blood type. Being an O-positive blood type, the presence of animal protein is very beneficial. Because of that, I have since re-introduced organic chicken, venison, elk and buffalo into "my eating habits."

For me, I have still chosen to eliminate all organic beef and dairy products; based on *The China Study*, written by T. Colin Campbell, PhD, and Thomas M. Campbell, MD. *Eat Right For Your Type*, by Dr. Peter J. D'Adamo, also recommends avoiding dairy products for O blood types as well as A blood types.

Physical & Mental Health

Exercise has also become a very important component of my new lifestyle. I started teaching yoga again in April, 2011. In addition to my yoga and meditation practice, which have always been a prominent part of my life, I felt it was important to incorporate weight training. My concern was entering into menopause at the age of 42 and the inability to take any medication to assist with this change. I have also become more in tune with "stressors" in my life, and proactively make choices that eliminate or at least help to reduce the occurrence of stress. Believe me; I'm happier and more content because of it. Joy flows through my body and mind. And I'm alive.

> *Joy flows through my body and mind. And I'm alive.*

Meal Plan

Meals are important. If you haven't before, you will now pay close attention to what is actually on the outside of a box in the grocery store. And seriously consider the following recommendations:

- Buy organic fruits and vegetables whenever possible.

- Become aware of monitoring the glycemic index of the fruits and vegetables you consume.
- Eat meals and snacks regularly throughout the day.
- Drink at least 48 ounces of filtered water a day.
- Drink 3-6 cups of green tea a day.
- Consume 3oz of organic animal protein at least 4 times a week. (For me, personally, I eat only organic chicken and wild game. The cow and pig are no longer an option.)
- Consume 2-3 servings of collard greens or kale a day.

I have invested in a juicer. I primarily juice vegetables on a regular basis. (Once again be conscious of the vegetable's sugar content.)

Sugar and processed foods have been removed from my meal plan. Natural sugars found in fruit are consumed in moderation along with a protein source. This helps to minimize a spike in sugar levels. Now, I know many of you may be thinking there is no way you can give up sugar. I'm here to tell you, it can be done.

Supplements and Vitamins

The following list of supplements and vitamins have been recommended by my naturopath.

Oncomar	Oncoplex	I-5 protein drink
Curcumin	DIM	COQ10
D3 4000UI	Cal/Mag	Triphala
Multivitamin	B-complex	Iron with C
Tumeric	Thiphala	Flax Oil

IV Vitamin C weekly (75,000 mg)

Eating healthy is time consuming and is not convenient by any stretch of the imagination. I don't want to fool you—it's my part-part time job! You can do it. You just need to have the desire and motivation if you want to regain and retain you health. Trying to prevent a recurrence of cancer was and is a strong motivator for me.

(Todd has been quite receptive to my new eating habits. He has actually incorporated some of these habits as well. Not only are we eating healthier together, we are creating new recipes together. The Gap has begun to close.)

Whole Foods Are Your Friends

My recommendation to you is to focus on as many "whole food" items as possible. Taking the time to read labels, will help you select healthier, more wholesome food choices. When shopping, buy fresh vegetables and fruits, nuts and seeds, whole grains sparingly, and only organic meats if you choose to eat meat. Stay away from packaged items. They are not your friend.

Don't be fooled by items just because they say "organic" or "healthy." Breakfast cereals are often quite misleading. Stick with organic steel cut oats—rolled oats has very little nutritional value. Add walnuts, cinnamon, fresh or frozen berries and almond or coconut milk as needed. You'd be surprised how wholesome and satisfying this is and delicious. Not only is cinnamon a wonderful spice to use in place of sugar, it also helps to reduce the glycemic index in foods. The next time you eat an apple, sprinkle some cinnamon on the slices. Go one step further; eat a handful of raw almonds along with your apple. You have a real treat in your mouth!

Preparation is key. In order to maintain successful eating habits, you need to plan and prepare some meals ahead of time. Making a large pot of soup at the beginning of your week will provide for a quick snack or meal. Additionally, hummus makes a wonderful snack and provides a good source of protein. Mix together almonds, pumpkin seeds and sunflower seeds; always keep a baggie in your car or purse.

Eating Out

Eating out will be the most challenging part of eating healthy. You mustn't be afraid to inform your server of your dietary restrictions. I have found many restaurants to be very accommodating. Even vacations can be enjoyable. I was pleasantly surprised how wonderful my dining experience was on Princess Cruise Line. The maitre d' and

I planned my meals each evening for the next day and made necessary modifications to meet my restrictions.

Todd and I also spent a week in Mexico and the concierge typed up a personalized letter in Spanish to alert my servers of my dietary restrictions. All I had to do was hand them the letter. They too were very accommodating.

I can only share with you some suggestions that I have done and learned along the way on my new food journey. It's been eye-opening to me, as I'm sure it will be to you. The bottom line is how determined and dedicated are you in doing everything within your control to try to prevent a recurrence of cancer?

You must take responsibility for your own health.

Dr. Steve Parcell's Take

I thought Luci would benefit from what I call wellness oncology to keep her cancer free. This includes testing nutrient levels, estrogen metabolites and immune function among other things. I thought she would benefit from IV vitamin C to kill off any malignant cells that were still in her body. The reasoning for this is as follows: Early clinical studies showed that high-dose vitamin C, given by intravenous and oral routes, may improve symptoms and prolong life in patients with cancer. Double-blind placebo-controlled studies of oral vitamin C therapy showed no benefit. Large doses (50-100g) given intravenously may result in plasma concentrations of about 25 times higher than can be achieved with the oral route. At these high concentrations, vitamin C is toxic to some cancer cells but not to normal cells.

High-dose injections of vitamin C, reduced tumor weight and growth rate by about 50 percent in mouse models of brain, ovarian, and pancreatic cancers, researchers from the national Institutes of health (NIH) report in the August 5, 2008 issue of The Proceedings of the National Academy of Sciences. The researchers traced Vitamins C anti-cancer effect to the formation of hydrogen peroxide in the extra-cellular fluid surrounding the tumors. Normal cells were unaffected.

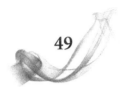

My Final Thoughts

For the Caregivers

We as fighters need your love and support as we have never needed it before. When we slip into a dark Moment, please help us to redirect our focus and energy to keep up the fight. Even though you are the caregiver, know it's okay for you to ask for help. What I have found from my experience was the overwhelming number of requests from friends offering to help. You just need to reach out. They are there—sometimes they don't know how to help—tell them.

For the Friends and Loved Ones

Everyone reacts differently to trauma and crisis. Don't be afraid to express your fears. It's okay. What is more difficult for a fighter is to have a friend totally disconnect themselves from our lives. For me personally, the unknown was harder to bear than if I would have been told of one's fear of hospitals.

Basic tasks and chores—ones we all take for granted—had become some of the greatest challenges for me during my chemo. Cooking, cleaning and laundry had become such a daunting task. If you are unsure of how to offer your assistance in such a way as to not feel as though you're imposing, make a meal or hire a cleaning service for your friend. These were just two of the many gestures I gratefully received from friends.

For the Physicians

Please don't let your ego get the better of you. While many of your diagnosing skills may come from a textbook, lecture or clinical trial, your most valuable resource may be right in front of you. Your patient. If there is only one point I hope to get across, it would be the importance of listening to the patient. For we know our bodies best. We do. And although you may think it's helpful, never, never, never give a patient a death sentence. Why would you want to paralyze your patient's ability to fight? As I said before, there is only One who knows this!

For the Fighter

What I have learned from this experience is the importance of keeping a positive outlook and mind-set. For me, prayer and meditation had a significant role in my recovery process. There is no doubt that you will have good days, bad days and perhaps some days that feel unbearable. You may also experience some alienation from friends. Perhaps the thought of seeing you ill or in a hospital is something they may not be able to face at this Moment. Try not to take it personally, for you do not know what might be going through their minds.

Surround yourself with both positive thoughts and people. You are not alone. You can get through this, but you must believe you can beat this, and you must have Faith.

Luci

Notes

Organizations

Cleaning For A Reason
A nonprofit organization partnering with maid services to offer free professional house cleanings to improve the lives of women undergoing cancer treatment.
www.CleaningForAReason.org

Colorado Ovarian Cancer Alliance (COCA)
The mission of the Colorado Ovarian Cancer Alliance (COCA) is to promote awareness about ovarian cancer through advocacy, education and support.
www.Colo-OvarianCancer.org

Jeanne Wallace, PhD, CNC (Nutritionist)
http://www.Nutritional-Solutions.net/LectureEvents.html

Life Spark Cancer Resources
Life Spark believes that a calm mind and a comfortable body can transform the cancer experience. Every day we provide gentle Reike and Healing Touch sessions to individuals with cancer because no one should go through cancer alone.
www.LifeSparkNow.org

Look Good … Feel Better
Look Good, Feel Better holds group workshops that teach beauty techniques to female cancer patients to help them combat the appearance-related side effects of cancer treatment.
www.LookGoodFeelBetter.org

Namaste Health Clinic
www.NamasteHealthCenter.com

National Ovarian Cancer Coalition (NOCC)
The mission of the NOCC is to raise awareness and promote education about ovarian cancer. The Coalition is committed to improving the survival rate and quality of life for women with ovarian cancer.
www.Ovarian.org

Natural Grocers
www.NaturalGrocers.com

Naturemed Clinic
"Bridging the gap" between alternative, holistic and conventional medicine. Offering Vitamin C IV therapy.
www.NaturemedClinic.com

Ovarian Cancer Support Group, founded by COCA
"Nicki's Circle" Ovarian Cancer Support Groups meet monthly around the Denver metro area and are open to anyone who has battled this disease. At meetings, we exchange information about ovarian cancer,

current medical research and how women can effectively advocate for obtaining the best health care possible. We also have the time and place to share the emotional ups and downs of this disease.
www.Colo-OvarianCancer.org/NickisCircle

Sunflower Markets
www.SunflowerMarkets.com

Tender Loving Care,
sponsored by the American Cancer Society
A not-for-profit website and catalog of the American Cancer Society. Our mission is to help women cope during and after cancer treatments by providing wigs and other hair loss products (plus how-to information) as well as mastectomy products.
www.TLCDirect.org

Whole Foods Market
www.WholeFoodsMarket.com

Recommended Books

D'Admano, Peter, *Eat Right For Your Type*, (New York: Berkley, 2002).

Fincher, Susanne F., *Coloring Mandalas for Insight, Healing and Self-Expression*, (Boston, Shambhala, 2000).

Singh Kaur, Artist/Author, *Crimson Collection Vol. 1 and 2*

T. Campbell, T. Colin, PhD, Thomas M. Campell II, *The China Study*, (Dallas: Ben Bella, 2006).

Yost, Debora, *The Anti-Cancer Food and Supplement Guide*, (New York: St. Martin's Press, 2010).

Articles

Alan Ames: *http://www.alanames.org/en/*.

Tara Parker-Pope, *New York Times*, November 12, 2009, *http://well.blogs.nytimes.com/2009/11/12/men-more-likely-to-leave-spouse-with-cancer/*.

About the Author

Luci Berardi is an ovarian cancer survivor, author and speaker. Luci was diagnosed in October, 2010 with Stage IV Ovarian Cancer. After going through a hysterectomy with de-bulking and the conventional regimen of chemotherapy, Luci remains cancer free. This journey 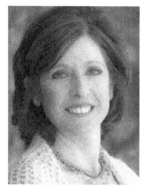 was the inspiration for Luci to write a book about her trials, mental state and triumph over this diagnosis. The use of conventional, alternative and spiritual therapies were paramount in her recovery. She provides hope and a renewal of Faith for the patient, the spouse and the family members and friends who walk a similar journey.

Luci is an advocate for raising awareness of this disease. She currently speaks to third-year medical students at the University of Colorado Health Sciences Department and for the Colorado Ovarian Cancer Alliance (COCA). She is also affiliated with Imerman Angels, a one-on-one cancer support network for other women in the depths of their own fight.

Bring Luci To You

Her story and the inspiration brought forth through her speaking engagements is ideal for any program that is focused on providing information, support and hope to women battling cancer and support to the ones that love them.

To inquire about having Luci speak at your organization, please submit a request at:

www.LuciBerardi.com

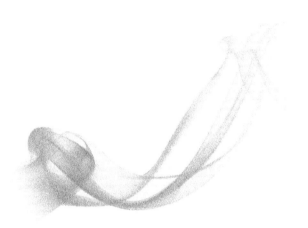